CONSCRIPTED TO CARE

Conscripted to Care

Women on the Frontlines
of the COVID-19 Response

JULIA SMITH

McGill-Queen's University Press
Montreal & Kingston · London · Chicago

© McGill-Queen's University Press 2023

ISBN 978-0-2280-1874-2 (cloth)
ISBN 978-0-2280-1875-9 (paper)
ISBN 978-0-2280-1931-2 (ePDF)
ISBN 978-0-2280-1932-9 (ePUB)

Legal deposit third quarter 2023
Bibliothèque nationale du Québec

Printed in Canada on acid-free paper that is 100% ancient forest free
(100% post-consumer recycled), processed chlorine free

This book has been published with the help of a grant from the Canadian Federation
for the Humanities and Social Sciences, through the Awards to Scholarly Publications
Program, using funds provided by the Social Sciences and Humanities Research
Council of Canada.

Publication has also been supported by the SFU University Publication Fund.

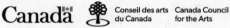

We acknowledge the support of the Canada Council for the Arts.

Nous remercions le Conseil des arts du Canada de son soutien.

Library and Archives Canada Cataloguing in Publication

Title: Conscripted to care: women on the frontlines of the COVID-19 response /
Julia Smith.

Names: Smith, Julia, 1981– author.

Description: Includes bibliographical references and index.

Identifiers: Canadiana (print) 20230201555 | Canadiana (ebook) 20230201598 |
ISBN 9780228018742 (cloth) | ISBN 9780228018759 (paper) |
ISBN 9780228019329 (ePUB) | ISBN 9780228019312 (ePDF)

Subjects: LCSH: Women—Canada—Social conditions—21st century. |
LCSH: Women—Canada—Economic conditions—21st century. | LCSH: Women
employees—Canada—Social conditions—21st century. | LCSH: Women employees—
Canada—Economic conditions—21st century. | LCSH: COVID-19 Pandemic,
2020—Social aspects—Canada. | LCSH: Equality—Health aspects—Canada. |
LCSH: Public health—Canada.

Classification: LCC HQ1453 .S65 2023 | DDC 305.420971—dc23

This book was typeset by Marquis Interscript in 10.5/13 Sabon.

Contents

Table and Figures

Acknowledgments

In writing this book, I've drawn on research conducted as part of the Gender and COVID-19 Project. It was through conversations with this broader team that I conceived of this book and refined my focus – thank you to all involved, especially for the motivation and encouragement during two particularly challenging years. In particular, I'm grateful to Clare Wenham for co-leading the overall project and Rosemary Morgan for co-leading the research with health-care workers. A small army of research assistants helped with data collection, analysis, and literature reviews. Thank you Alexander Korzuchowski, Christina Memmott, Alice Mũrage, Heang-Lee Tan, and Niki Oveisi. And of course, none of this work would have been possible without research funding from the Canadian Institutes of Health Research and BC Women's Health Foundation.

As a working mother, other people's labour enabled me to have the time necessary to write this book, during a period when time was in particularly short supply. I relied on the wonderful educators at the SFU Childcare Society to provide quality consistent care to my kid. My partner took on extra care work at home and my parents filled in childcare gaps – thank you all.

And most important, thank you to the women who shared the experiences that fill the following pages. Thank you for giving up time you didn't have, for expending that much more emotional energy to share your lives with a stranger, for giving your expertise and knowledge so generously. Thank you for taking care of so many of us and our loved ones throughout the pandemic – this book is for you.

CONSCRIPTED TO CARE

1

Introduction

Women are being conscripted into this. They're being drafted,
but unlike the soldiers in the Second World War who got paid, pensions,
and training, women's sacrifice isn't acknowledged. It's just expected.

Key informant

I remember the day COVID-19 became a reality for me. I had just left
a relative's seventieth birthday party and was standing on a beach
looking out over the Strait of Georgia in British Columbia (BC),
Canada. It was one of those March days when it's almost warm in the
sun but freezing in the shade. Just as I was about to get back into
the car with my family, my sister, a physician, called and said case
numbers were increasing, and I might want to keep my three-year-old
child home from daycare. I called my parents and made plans to visit,
so they could help with child care while my partner and I worked
from their basement – both of us being privileged to be able to
work from home. We thought we would be there for a week or two.
We ended up staying for three months. During those initial months,
I, together with a remarkable team of researchers from around the
world, began the Gender and COVID-19 Project.

We had all done some research on gender and health crises, so we
knew that women were the ones most often disproportionately affected,
in a myriad of ways, but that work had been difficult because of a lack of
data. For example, during the West African Ebola outbreak of 2014–16,
evidence of gender differences in morbidity and mortality was spotty
and contradictory (Wenham, Smith, and Morgan 2020). When we
reviewed academic publications on both the Ebola and Zika outbreaks,

we found that only 1 per cent of articles mentioned women or gender (Davies and Bennett 2016). Another review found only twelve articles, published between 2010 and 2019, on the experiences of women health-care workers during crises (Morgan et al. 2022). We decided this time would be different; we would collect the data and do real-time gender analysis so that there would be no excuse for ignoring the unequal effects of the unfolding pandemic.

My own research, through a convergence of coincidences and inter-ests, focused on women working in essential roles in the health and education sectors. A year into the pandemic, I realized I had spoken with over 200 women engaged in frontline work via interviews and focus groups. Recognizing the wealth of knowledge and experience contained in their accounts, and fearful it could be lost in the desire to return to "normal," motivated me to compile and share their stories in this book. My aim in writing it is to amplify the experiences of women working on the front lines of the COVID-19 response during the first year of the pandemic as a unique contribution to Canada's collective memory of the pandemic. My hope is that the analysis will inform a more equitable pandemic response, recovery, and prepared-ness, from which others can draw to advance our understanding of the gendered effects of health crises.

Over the past two years, my research, and that of the Gender and COVID-19 Project, has become part of a larger movement to centre gender within the COVID-19 response. It has been inspiring to see the literature grow on the differential gendered effects of the pandemic. Between January 2020 and January 2021, sixty-four articles were published on women healthcare workers and COVID-19 (Morgan et al. 2022). UN Women, United Nations Development Programme (UNDP), and Global Health 50/50 compiled datasets of gender-desegregated data and gender-sensitive policy responses (UNDP 2022). Civil society organizations, such as Feminists Deliver, and the media reported on childcare challenges and lack of access to gender-affirming surgeries, among other issues. During the first few months of the pandemic, media outlets called me almost daily and peppered me with questions about the pandemic's effects on women's employment, security, and well-being. Feminist organizations published recovery plans as early as June 2020, influencing the Canadian federal government to set out its own feminist response to COVID-19 in the September 2020 budget statement (Government of Canada 2020). For a moment, perhaps about five months into the pandemic, when the first wave had subsided and the second hadn't started, I had hope that, this time, the pandemic response and recovery would be different, that we would indeed "#buildbackbetter."

I'm writing this in March 2022, my optimism dimmed but not exhausted. The Gender and COVID-19 Project, which I co-lead, and other initiatives are still documenting the effects of ongoing waves of the pandemic and providing rapid policy analysis from the local to the global level. Civil society organizations are campaigning for greater investments in care infrastructure to address many of the effects of the pandemic on women, and every now and then the media runs a story about how stressed out parents or healthcare workers are. But none of it seems to have held back the tide of unequal effects borne by women and other equity-deserving groups. For example:

- Canada is one of the few countries with more cases of COVID among women than men, and where more women than men have died from COVID-related causes. This is likely due to the combination of the number of women living in long-term care, where the majority of outbreaks have occurred, and the dominance of women in frontline work (Berry et al. 2020).
- Canada's proportion of healthcare workers, over 80 per cent of whom are women, as a share of its total COVID-19 cases (94,811 cases/6.8 per cent) was higher one year into the pandemic than comparable countries such as France, Germany, and the United States (CIHI 2021a).
- Of those made unemployed during the initial months of the pandemic, 58 per cent were women (despite making up just 48 per cent of the workforce), and it took thirteen months for women's employment to reach pre-pandemic levels, compared with just six months for men (Shrma and Smith 2021).
- Reports of domestic violence increased during the initial months of the pandemic, with a Vancouver crisis line reporting a 300 per cent increase in April 2020 (Daya and Azpiri 2020).
- In July 2020, 71 per cent of women reported increased depression, stress, and anxiety because of increased COVID-19-related care burdens (Oxfam Canada 2020).

These statistics are a reminder that despite unprecedented attention to the gendered effects of COVID-19, inequities have continued to unfold in starkly predictable patterns.

This contrast – between increased gender rhetoric and persistent unequal outcomes – demands a critical analysis of why and how gender-based analysis has been incorporated into the COVID-19 response. In her article "Threat Not Solution," Harman (2021) explains the rise in attention to gender inequality and COVID-19 as the result not only of sustained advocacy from feminist groups, but also of the fact that this is one of the first pandemics to affect women in high-income countries, such as Canada, and women from higher socioeconomic classes. Harman suggests that, as a result, gender-based responses are less about challenging current power hierarchies than maintaining them, raising important questions about how gender is framed within the COVID-19 response, noting that it is only prioritized "when gender becomes a solution to the crisis – for example, by assuming gender norms that women will home-school their children" (Harman 2021). In contrast, the effects of such work on women are rarely recognized: "The threat the same gender norms represent to women's health and wellbeing – that the burden of managing home-schooling, work and psycho-social family support during the pandemic gives women little time to prioritize their own health, will damage their mental and physical wellbeing … is seen as less relevant" (Harman 2021). Recognizing this tension, this book aims to document the experiences of women on the front lines both in terms of the invaluable contributions they have made to the COVID-19 response – honouring their power and fortitude – and identifying the structures that have downloaded the responsibility to respond on to women without corresponding support, assuming women will bear the costs – as they have indeed done.

THE CANADIAN COVID-19 CONTEXT

Canada is held up neither as an example of an exceptional COVID-19 response nor a failed one. In terms of mortality and case numbers (37,240 deaths and 3.4 million cases as of March 2022), it fared better than its southern neighbour, but not as well as many European countries (Our World Data 2022). The overall response to COVID-19 in Canada, and BC, reflected a "balanced-containment" approach, similar to many other OECD (Organisation for Economic Co-operation and Development) states, characterized by attempts to balance primary health effects (cases, hospitalizations, and deaths) and the economic and social disruptions caused by infection control measures (Oliu-Barton et al. 2021). There are and will continue to be numerous analyses of how this strategy has played out, so I will not assess that here.

The national response to COVID-19 and the provincial responses within it have rolled with the waves of the pandemic, what was known at the time, and the political and economic context. Across the country, the initial months of the pandemic (March to June 2020) were characterized by lockdown, with most services and schools closed due to fears of overwhelming hospitals, as information about transmission and severity was still emerging. As businesseses shuttered and industries such as tourism ground to a halt, the federal government introduced the Canada Emergency Response Benefit (CERB), providing $2,000 a month to those who had lost work due to COVID-19, as well as numerous initiatives to support businesses. The summer of 2020 provided a moment of false hope, social gatherings, and "recovery" plans. But by the fall, a second wave had cancelled Thanksgiving and then Christmas gatherings. CERB was revamped into the Canada Recovery Benefit, paid sick and care days were legislated for COVID-19-related absences, efforts were made to ensure that schools and child care stayed open, while restrictions remained on restaurants, gyms, and other businesses where people gathered. Most of us spent much of the winter of 2020–21 in our immediate-family bubbles, still working remotely and avoiding unnecessary travel. Cases peaked again in the spring of 2021, but the vaccine roll-out provided hope that the curve would again bend downwards. Restrictions eased as cases fell during the summer of 2021. The content of this book is situated within this first year of the pandemic, with a specific focus on the time period of each chapter (see table 1.1). Each wave and ebb of infection, response, and hope directly affected the women whose stories are included here.

The COVID-19 response must also be situated in the broader health context, because COVID-19 was layered onto previous crises. BC, in particular, continues to experience an opioid epidemic, with 2,200 people dying due to toxic drugs in 2020 – a 26 per cent increase from the previous year (BC Coroners Service 2021). COVID-19 interacted with this epidemic as border restrictions contributed to the presence of toxic drugs, pandemic-related stress led to increased harmful-substance use, and physical distancing requirements forced many people to use substances alone. The disruption in community-based services during the initial lockdown cut off many, already experiencing multiple vulnerabilities, from their support networks. This interlinked pandemic occurred in a context of rising housing and overall living costs, again exacerbated by COVID-19-related unemployment and supply-chain disruptions. As has been well-documented elsewhere, COVID-19 exacerbated many pre-existing social determinants of health (Abrams and Szefler 2020). It is these effects that many of the women in the following chapters were responding to, both personally and professionally, before and during COVID, with the pandemic adding another layer of crisis.

When it comes to considering the gendered effects of the pandemic, Canada often comes out at the top of the list. An early assessment by Care International and ongoing monitoring by UNDP and UN Women lists Canada as one of the countries with the highest number of gender-sensitive measures within its COVID-19 response (UNDP 2022; CARE Canada 2020). Including gender considerations reflects the federal government's long-standing commitment to Gender-Based Analysis Plus (GBA+). Overseen by Women and Gender Equality Canada, GBA+ aims to ensure that gender and intersecting inequities are taken into consideration when developing, implementing, and monitoring policy (Women and Gender Equality Canada 2022). Since its inception in 2011, the concept and application of GBA+ have been both celebrated and widely criticized, and have remained a persistent feature in Canadian policymaking (Christoffersen and Hankivsky 2021). Following a 2016 report from the Auditor General of Canada, which indicated the need to implement GBA+ more fully across government sectors, Women and Gender Equality Canada developed a four-year Action Plan on GBA+ (2016–20) that included commitments to develop new GBA+ tools, required training for civil servants, and instituted mandatory GBA+ policy assessments. This has resulted in almost all COVID-19 policies undergoing GBA+ assessments and commitments from the federal government to address the secondary effects of the pandemic on women and other equity-deserving groups. As a result, Canada's example provides a critical case study to understand the possibilities and limits of attempts to address the unequal effects of a health crisis on women.

Within Canada's federal system, provincial governments have jurisdiction over most economic, health, and social policy. BC, where all but one chapter of this book is set, has also committed to a GBA+ approach to policy development. In 2018, the BC government committed to "ensure gender equality is reflected in all budgets, policies and programs" (Office of the Premier 2018) and created a Gender Equity Office within the Ministry of Finance. However, little information is publicly available about how the government is applying GBA+ and it is only occasionally mentioned in budgets and other fiscal documents. Similar to what has been observed at the federal level, provincial progress toward incorporating GBA+ and taking requisite policy action has been mixed. Cameron and Tedds (2020) note that the BC government has been complicit in the systems that construct the inequities GBA+ seeks to rectify, such as those that have created a housing and childcare crisis in much of the province. Civil society report cards note that women and gender-diverse individuals from the most vulnerable groups, such as sex workers, were particularly left behind by COVID-19 response policies (Sproule and Prochuk 2020). Despite these well-documented limitations of federal and provincial GBA+ approaches, Canada and BC are unique in their commitment to consider intersectional gender inequities within their responses to the pandemic. What can be learned from such attempts and how can they be strengthened?

A GENDER ANALYSIS OF WOMEN'S EXPERIENCES

This book is about women, who I define as anyone who identifies as such regardless of what sex they were assigned at birth. I apply this broad definition recognizing that "woman" is a socially constructed category defined by gender norms and roles. Gender roles include tasks and behaviour deemed appropriate and expected of a particular gender both at work and at home. As Butler notes, individuals "do gender" by repeating specific tasks and acting out norms (Butler 2020). It is through these performative acts that they identify with a gender construct and that others recognize and label their gender. This book focuses on those who "do" what is associated, in Canada, with the gender defined as "woman." It further argues that these gendered acts and expectations have placed women in roles essential to the COVID-19 response.

Expectations about how women in essential roles respond to the pandemic are structured by gender norms, the often unspoken rules that govern the attributes valued and considered acceptable for a particular gender. Gender norms not only affect individual behaviour, but are embedded in institutions, including our homes, workplaces, and government, defining who occupies leadership positions, whose contributions are valued, and whose needs are accommodated (Morgan et al. 2016). Gender-based analysis seeks to make these roles and norms explicit and identify gender bias within policies and processes that favour or reflect the interests of one or some genders over others (Elson 2010). In this book, I apply gender analysis to understand how roles and norms have structured women's experiences of the pandemic and how they have, in turn, reinforced or resisted these structures.

I recognize that the focus on women, while including trans women, limits the gender analysis in that it does not include the experiences of those who identify as two-spirit, non-binary, gender diverse, trans men, or men. By no means do I intend to deny the experiences of those engaged in essential work who do not identify as women or suggest that the parenting and related care work challenges described in these chapters only apply to women. There is a need for research that documents the full range of gendered experiences of COVID-19, particularly of people, often rendered invisible, who identify outside the man-woman dichotomy. Still, this book's contribution is to amplify women's experiences while illuminating the gendered constructs that shape these and others' experiences of the pandemic. I hope it will be one contribution among many that will enable a deeper understanding of how gender constructs have shaped the response to COVID-19.

I further recognize that gender identity intersects with additional social positions related to race, sexuality, ethnicity, (dis)ability and socioeconomic status. Intersectional analysis is incorporated in this book by emphasizing women's multiple and overlapping identities and is applied to prioritize the experiences of those women most affected by school and childcare closures. For example, the chapter on moms includes a specific focus on the moms of children with special needs as a group highly affected by school and childcare closures. The chapter on childcare educators emphasizes the challenges faced by racialized and newcomer educators, who make up a large portion of that workforce. While integrating intersectional analysis, I recognize that the primary focus on women's gendered experiences highlights specific experiences over others, which may overshadow other structural inequities. In particular, most of the participants in the research that informs this book are settlers, with just five of the 214 participants identifying as Indigenous. It is important to recognize the colonial backdrop to the context of COVID-19 in Canada, and I urge readers to seek out Indigenous accounts and analyses of the COVID-19 response, such as the work done by the Yellowhead Institute (yellowheadinstitute.org). This book acknowledges that the specific focus on gender is a limitation while contending that gender analysis directs attention to what those on the front lines of the COVID-19 response are most likely to have in common – that over 80 per cent of essential workers identify as women.

ON BEING "CONSCRIPTED"

I came up with the title of this book while reading the transcript of an interview with a key informant from a labour organization. She said, "Women are being conscripted into this. They're being drafted, but unlike the soldiers in the Second World War who got paid, pensions, and training, women's sacrifice isn't acknowledged. It's just expected." I was instantly reminded of how Canadian culture has conferred hero status on soldiers who fought in the First and Second World War and the social support programs introduced following the Second World War that largely benefited the returning soldiers. I also remembered how my grandfather, a veteran who had landed on the beaches of Normandy on D-Day during the Second World War, shrugged off any conflating of war and heroism. He did not attend Remembrance Day ceremonies because he said there was nothing good to remember, just wet socks, lost friends, and getting in trouble for stealing the officers' rum. I also thought about my Granny, who, during the war, got an office job with the federal government for a brief time but had to go back to cleaning houses when the men returned. Her contributions were never recognized, whereas my grandfather wished his had been ignored.

It is these contradictions that I aim to highlight by using military terms such as conscripted and front lines. I recognize that many feminists reject the use of military language because they see it as reinforcing the violence that has been used to oppress women and assert the "dominant voice of militarized masculinity" (Cohn 1987). Invoking military language can be viewed as perpetuating narratives that justify violence and make heroes out of those who perpetrated it (Warren and Cady 1994). As Simone de Beauvoir writes of Western militarized culture, "It is not in giving life but in risking life that man is raised above the animal: that is why superiority has been accorded

in humanity not to the sex that brings forth but to that which kills"
(1949, 800); in other words, killing by men is positioned as superior
to caring by women. Consequently, many argue that military language
cannot be used to dismantle patriarchal norms and systems. I argue
that in appropriating such language, not only is it possible to capitalize
on its power but also to expose its contradictions.

For example, within the COVID-19 response, women have been
both celebrated as heroes and saddled with increased drudgery. They
have been both honoured and threatened for providing essential
services, such as vaccinations. They have seen demand for their labour
increase while supports decrease. The women whose stories are
included here stepped up to the challenge posed by COVID-19
willingly and often with vigour – much like the images of those young
Canadian men lining up to enlist in a horrific conflict. And, much like
those men, it was less a choice, and more a duty, and impossible for
them to know what they were signing up for ahead of time. Now
writing this, two years after the initial public health emergency
announcement, it is clear that many women on the front lines have
suffered for their commitment; the question is, has their contribution
been recognized, honoured, and indemnified?

TO CARE

As indicated in the title, this book is also about care – health care,
child care, elder care, and the care provided to those who are sick,
tired, hungry, sad, and lonely. Care involves maintaining the world
of and meeting the needs of others. We care for others and ourselves
when we help satisfy the basic biological needs necessary for survival
and basic functioning, relieve suffering or pain, and develop or sustain
basic capabilities for engaging in society, learning, and caring for
others. Caring makes the development and basic well-being of another
its direct end. It produces and reproduces society by providing
citizens, workers, voters, consumers, students, and all the others who
populate its institutions (Braedley and Luxton 2021). Care is not only
interactive and communicative; it transforms social relations
(Habermas 1987).

A feminist ethic of care argues that there is moral significance in the
fundamental elements of relationships and dependencies in human
life, and that the "ethic of care" associated with women should be as
valued and esteemed as the "ethic of rights" embedded in Western

liberal philosophy (primarily written by and about men) that justifies the claims individuals can make on others and on society (such as the right to liberty) (Gilligan, Ward, and Taylor 1988; Gilligan 2016). Care theory points out that most Western philosophers have ignored how central to human relations is the motivation to care and be cared for. Baier (1985) argues that moral theories, such as liberalism, that do not give proper moral recognition to caring display a form of bad faith, since caring forms the necessary ground of all moral practices and sustains these practices across generations. Such arguments point out that caretaking work creates a collective or societal debt that obligates all members of society to support and contribute to caring activities to reflect its broad social value (Fineman 2001). Failure to assume and pay this debt, for example by not investing in care infrastructure, is "at best churlish, at worst manifestly unjust" since caring forms the foundation of society and is central to the quality of all of our lives (Baier 1985, 30).

Feminist political economy (FPE) situates this debt within social, economic, and political contexts, recognizing that who does what care work, under what types of conditions, is shaped by dominant neoliberal policy paradigms. FPE analyzes the intersections of formal and informal labour, divisions of labour, matters of gender and race, and conditions of work. It points out that in much of the world, including Canada, paid care work remains undervalued, female dominated, low status, and poorly paid. This is the result of gender bias that portrays care work as something requiring few skills that all women and girls are inherently able to do (Esplen 2009). In Canada, caring professions are dominated by women, including a disproportionate number of racialized women, whose work is often precarious (Vosko and Zukewich 2003). Poor pay and work conditions are enforced by exploiting the personal relationships and emotional connections embedded in care work, discouraging workers from taking job action that might threaten the well-being of those they care for. As Folbre writes: "Care workers become, in a sense, prisoners of love" (2008, 376). So, while the undervaluing of care work and the failure to see it as a profession are used to justify policies that neglect or ignore those providing care, the exploitation of the emotional bonds inherent in such work inhibits care workers from demanding change.

Unpaid care work, similar to paid care work, is embedded in feelings of moral obligation and commitment to others' well-being.

It has both benefits – in terms of strong family and community ties and quality of service to dependents – and costs – in terms of resources required, lost opportunities, and forgone wages (Rai and Waylen 2013). Policy environments and gender norms structure the relationship between these costs and benefits, as well as who pays for and who earns from them, with the majority of unpaid care work completed by women at their own cost for the benefit of others. Economic production and trade would not be possible without unpaid care work, which ensures basic needs and develops the basic capabilities of future workers. When states shed responsibilities for social protections, such as child care, unpaid care work is further shifted onto women, with little recognition of this downstream effect or any effort to understand that those increased costs should be mitigated. Unpaid care work is often expected to fill gaps in or subsidize the public sector's provisioning of services.

Antonopoulos presents a useful conceptualization of the relationships between unpaid care, paid care, and productive labour within the circle of care (Antonopoulos 2008). The circle of care (see figure 1.1) demonstrates how the conditions, provisions, and accessibility of paid care work directly affect the level, distribution, and conditions of unpaid care, which, in turn, affect women's opportunities to enter and remain in paid work, all of which influence outcomes for care recipients. It suggests that to understand, for example, a gender wage gap, the availability of paid care also needs to be considered, as do gender roles in unpaid care and paid work. Similarly, questions regarding why women continue to do the majority of unpaid care must be situated within discussions of gender discrimination in paid work and accessibility to paid care services. The circle demonstrates the necessity of not only analyzing effects within sectors of the circle (for example, the effect of the pandemic on women's participation in the labour force) but also on the relationships between sectors and how changes in one sector affect another.

The COVID-19 pandemic provides an opportunity to explore these relationships as the care economy has been shocked by closures and interruptions in paid care, with notable gendered effects on unpaid care. Along with the rest of the economy, the circle of care has been shocked by the pandemic, and policy choices have structured who absorbs these shocks and at what cost. The women in this book are at the heart of this crisis as those who provide both paid and unpaid care.

Levels and distribution of unpaid care affect
conditions of unpaid care work and care
workers' ability to participate in other paid work

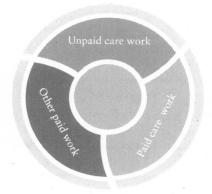

Lack of gender
equality in labour
market, gender
pay gap, working
conditions etc.
affects outcomes
of care

Supply and working
conditions of care
workers affect their
ability to do other
paid work and how
they distribute time
for unpaid care work

Figure 1.1 The circle of care

APPROACH AND METHODS

The experiences shared in this book are not meant to be generalizable
or representative of the experiences of all women engaged in frontline
work or even the professions discussed here. Instead, I adopt a lived
experience approach rooted in a commitment to creating knowledge
grounded in the experiences of people belonging to the groups most
affected by the subject of the research, recognizing that knowledge is
gained by acknowledging the specificity and uniqueness of lives, rather
than by simply adding or counting women (Yarrow and Pagan 2020).
The chapters that follow focus on everyday life occurrences to capture
both the "ordinary" and the "extraordinary" across a range of women
who are in a comparably similar situation: responding to the COVID-19
pandemic. While recognizing that each experience is unique, elements
of commonality facilitate an analysis of clusters of shared experiences,
illustrating recurring patterns, and instances of struggle and empowerment (McIntosh and Wright 2019). Such scholarship aims to make
visible experiences that are often ignored to illustrate both how policies
structure contexts and how agency is exercised within them. The
holders of these experiences, as those with intimate knowledge, are
then recognized as experts, particularly in evaluating the effects of
pandemic response on the women who staffed it.

To gather such lived expertise, over the first fifteen months of the COVID-19 pandemic (March 2020 to June 2021) I conducted focus groups and semi-structured interviews with 182 women (table 1.1) working on the front lines of the COVID-19 response, and eighteen key informants representing civil society organizations engaged in women's rights work or representing essential workers. These key informants represented national advocacy organizations and local service delivery organizations – and everything in between. They provided insight into the participants' broader context. The timing and context of data collection are always important, particularly during a pandemic, since perspectives and experiences reflect waves of infection, what was known about the virus, and policy decisions at the time. Therefore, each chapter should be read with its time frame in mind.

Focus group and interview participants were recruited through advertisements emailed and disseminated through unions, professional associations, and women's groups. Because some of this research was conducted in partnership with organizations such as BC Women's Health Foundation and the Alberta Teachers' Association, these organizations disseminated calls for participants, as did a number of allied civil society organizations – all of whom I am indebted to for their support. Conversations with these partners also helped inform the overall methodology and interview and focus group guides, as well as the preliminary analysis. Inclusion criteria for participants of focus groups and semi-structured interviews included self-identifying as a woman, being nineteen years old or older, being engaged in paid frontline work, or being a parent. Because of the physical distancing requirements of the pandemic, focus groups and interviews were held virtually through Zoom and lasted about one hour. I conducted the vast majority of interviews and focus groups, with other team members, to whom I am also indebted, conducting a handful. All focus groups and interviews, except those with physicians, were audio-recorded and then transcribed. The focus groups and interviews were semi-structured, with a mix of questions and discussions. Simon Fraser University provided ethical approval for this research, and participants provided informed consent for their data to be presented anonymously in outputs such as this book.

As much of this research was conducted under the umbrella of the Gender and COVID-19 Project, I first analyzed much data for more immediate outputs with a team (to whom I am also indebted) drawing

Table 1.1
Research participants

Who	When	Where	How	Number
Physicians	June to September 2020	Vancouver, BC	Four focus groups	27
Early Childhood Educators	May to September 2020	Lower Mainland of BC	Interviews	9
Moms	May 2020 to May 2021	Lower Mainland of BC	Interviews	27
Midwives	December 2020 to February 2021	BC	Interviews and three focus groups	13
LTC workers	February to April 2021	BC	Interviews and five focus groups	27
Nurses	February to March 2021	BC	Interviews and four focus groups	14
Community health and social care workers	March to April 2021	BC	Interviews and four focus groups	26
Teachers	March to June 2021	Alberta	Interviews and five focus groups	39

on framework and applied thematic analysis approaches (Guest, MacQueen, and Namey 2014; Gale et al. 2013). Preliminary results and early publications were shared back to partner organizations, and those participants who indicated interest, through discussions and briefs, with feedback gratefully incorporated. Through this process, I developed the core themes of this book, noticing similarities across professions and experiences. I then revisited the data independently, through a more reflexive thematic approach (Braun and Clarke 2014), to construct codes within these themes, map their relationships, and reflect on patterns and differences. The process of revisiting the data multiple times and for varying purposes generated a rich reflective approach.

Conducting research during a pandemic means building the ship while it is sailing. That requires humility. Holding interviews and focus groups remotely prevented the type of relationship-building, participant observation, and more in-depth methods common in feminist research, which I previously preferred and was most familiar with. As a result, I learned many lessons in the process of conducting this research. For example, following the initial focus groups and interviews, I realized that greater wellness support was required for participants (and me). I solicited the services of a professional counselling company that provided resources to be shared with participants and availed focus group participants of a counsellor in a separate Zoom room for them to access. Noting that focus groups of healthcare workers did not initially reflect the diversity within the field, I ensured, for the focus groups with teachers, that there was a group specifically for Indigenous and racialized women, with facilitators who identified as racialized women. I used semi-structured interviews and purposive sampling to gain perspectives from women from a range of ethnicities, backgrounds, geographies, and socioeconomic contexts. Yet, as noted above, by no means does this book claim to represent a full spectrum of experiences of the gendered nature of frontline work. Instead, it aims to share illustrative lived experiences as one window into the pandemic response.

A PERSONAL REFLECTION

I heard the experiences contained in this book over Zoom or the phone from a secluded office. Most of the time, my kid was with my parents or in a wonderful childcare centre, my partner was working from home (hopefully doing laundry and prepping dinner), and when I felt anxious, I would go for walks in the forest around the university. As a white, middle-class, partnered, cisgender woman, my privilege mitigated the risk and hardships associated with the pandemic. In contrast, the women I spoke to were exposed daily to the risk of infection, alongside racism, stigma, trauma, and other threats. Most experienced challenges accessing paid child care, and many did not have partners or social networks to rely on. This difference is important to acknowledge because, while these women graciously gave me their time and permission to share their stories, what I recount here is my interpretation of their lived experience. I am at risk of the privilege hazard: "the phenomenon that makes those who occupy the most privileged positions among us – those with good educations, respected credentials, and professional accolades – so poorly equipped to recognize instances of oppression in the world" (D'Ignazio and Klein 2020). My lack of a lived experience similar to that of those who participated in this research inhibits my ability to fully comprehend their experiences, particularly harms they have experienced or might experience because of inequities, and to imagine possible solutions.

I have aimed to mitigate this hazard and honour the experiences shared by conducting research in a way that enabled participants to lead and share as much or as little as they wished on topics important to them. I did this through a semi-structured approach to qualitative research based on exploring themes rather than asking specific questions and being flexible in the direction of the research. As I produced research briefs and articles, I shared them with participants and invited feedback. Each chapter's conclusion includes participants' recommendations on how the challenges they experienced might be overcome in both practical and immediate and longer-term systemic change. This is an imperfect process, but I have aimed to tell the stories here with humility and the goal of amplifying the voices of those most affected. Recognizing that with privilege comes responsibility, the aim of this book is not just academic (to produce new knowledge) but also normative (to inform and advocate for change).

I further recognize that this analysis remains influenced by my bias. I am not an essential frontline worker, but, like so many of us, I have many essential workers among my family and friends. I feel grateful for the wonderful early childcare educators who take care of my kid as I write this book. A brilliant midwife attended her birth. These experiences no doubt influence my analysis, particularly in making me sympathetic to the struggles faced by the women I spoke with and being grateful for their service. I admit this bias, including personal anecdotes in some chapters, and argue that it enables me to have a deep, if still limited, understanding of the experiences shared here.

THE STRUCTURE
AND THEMES OF THE BOOK

The following chapters focus on the experiences of women working in specific sectors, some of which are frequently associated within pandemic responses, such as nursing and medicine, and others that are more often ignored, such as midwifery and early childhood education. I have tried to order and alternate chapters to avoid reproducing hierarchies that value contributions based on pay or social status. Therefore, chapters jump from well-recognized healthcare roles to the less celebrated roles, including those outside of public health such as education and child care. My hope is that this structure will map the diversity of women's contributions to pandemic response – though I do also recognize that many essential roles, such as food service and delivery, are not focused on here.

As you read each chapter, it is important to remember the timing of the research. Interviews and focus groups conducted during the early months of the pandemic reflect experiences in a context of extreme information uncertainty, while later data collection occurred alongside the vaccine roll-out. The waves of COVID-19 infections have been juxtaposed with waves of hope that the pandemic was ending, and that the situation would improve. As I finish this manuscript, public health leaders are telling us to get used to living with the virus. By the time you read this, I am sure further developments will have shaken our assumptions about COVID-19, and pandemics more broadly. As you read, please consider what it was like during that first year of COVID-19 as these women staffed the front lines at work and at home.

As noted above, the contents of this book are drawn from a number of sub-projects under the umbrella of the broader Gender and COVID-19 Project. As I was speaking with nurses and teachers, mothers, and long-term-care workers, I was struck as much by the similarities as the differences between their experiences. As I began to map patterns, I realized that what was common across the accounts was not the women's experiences, which are often unique, but the gender norms, roles, and institutional forms that structure them. Women's experiences, while differing in particulars and severity, were similarly shaped by pre-existing gender inequities, which COVID-19, in classic vicious-cycle fashion, exacerbated. Concurrently, and somewhat contradictorily, the pandemic, as an extraordinary event, created an opportunity for change, which women and other equity-deserving groups have seized. The chapter sections reflect these common themes:

- the *quadruple burden* placed upon women, i.e., the triple burden of unpaid care, paid employment, and household/community management alongside emotional labour;
- the opportunities and restrictions, celebrations and contradictions that came with the label of *being essential* – or not;
- the effects on *mental health*, such as *moral distress and burnout*, among essential workers; and
- how *power* has been exercised within the response to shape and resist gendered structures of oppression.

The Quadruple Burden

The concept of the triple burden refers to the responsibilities placed on women in most neoliberal economies to complete paid work and unpaid care work, and manage family or community relationships. While gender roles have shifted over time, resulting in an increase in women in the paid workforce in Canada – from 24 per cent in 1953 to 64.7 per cent in 2019 – men's participation in unpaid labour inside the home has not adapted to a corresponding degree, with women still doing two to three times the amount of unpaid care work compared with men (Statistics Canada 2018). Women's multiple responsibilities have wide-ranging effects. Bryson and Deery describe how gender inequalities are sustained by differences in the use and experience of time among men and women and "that 'time cultures' are bound up with power and control" (2010, 91). Men have, on average, more control over their time outside work than women, with family members laying more claims on women's time. Women feel more rushed in their daily lives and are more likely to be expected to attend to household work. This uneven burden restricts women's earning potential and professional and personal development and has negative health effects (Hjálmsdóttir, Bjarnadóttir, and Eðvarðs Sigurðssonar 2021)

Not all the unpaid work women do in the home and for their families or communities is physical. As Schwarzenbach writes, caring includes "all those rational activities (thinking about particular others and their needs, caring for them, cooking their meals, etc.) which go towards reproducing a particular set of relationships between persons over time" (1996, 102). In heterosexual couples, mothers are much more likely to be household managers than fathers (Ciciolla and Luthar 2019). Their work includes the mental burden that goes into planning, decision-making, and monitoring family and community members to ensure they have what they need. A key characteristic of such work is that it is challenging to delegate, because delegation by definition requires management work – asking a spouse to make an appointment for a child can be almost as much or more work than doing it oneself. Mental work often goes unnoticed by other family members, as do the effects on the mother's well-being, such as stress and anxiety (Dean, Churchill, and Ruppanner 2022).

In addition, women are more likely than men to take on emotional labour at home and at work. Emotional labour refers to activities affecting the emotional well-being of other family members and the provision of emotional support (Curran et al. 2015). A key aspect of emotional labour is managing one's own emotions to be able to provide support to another (Gray 2009). Substantial research has demonstrated that emotional labour is gendered in that it is most often expected of women and often becomes part of women's routines. Emotional labour has traditionally been identified with women's work and the role of the mother in the family. The portrayal of emotional labour as a "natural activity" for women has resulted in it being devalued culturally and economically (Dean, Churchill, and Ruppanner 2022). Such devaluations also result in a lack of recognition of emotional labour conducted in professional settings. Health systems research has documented how women healthcare workers take on more emotional labour in patient care, partly due to gender norms and partly due to the gendered composition of the healthcare workforce, but are paid less (Gray 2009). Emotional labour costs time, increases women's mental load, and can negatively affect women's emotional and mental well-being. Due to the numerous accounts of the burden of emotional labour shared by women essential workers, I have expanded the concept of the triple burden to also include this work, and describe a quadruple burden.

All four burdens – paid work, unpaid care, household and community management, and emotional labour – were dramatically increased by COVID-19, as will be demonstrated in the following chapters. Each chapter starts with a section on the quadruple burden, looking first at how gendered work burdens in the paid environment changed in response to COVID-19. While these changes were often sector-wide, so not specific to women's experiences – because most of the workplaces described here (all except those of physicians) are feminized – their effects reflect how the feminization of care-related work results in work or conditions that are under-resourced, poorly supported, and often inadequately paid. The analysis then turns to the additional burdens that were layered on top of paid care work, such as unpaid child and elder care, analyzing the relationships between types of responsibility and the strategies women employed to meet the needs of patients, clients, children, family, and colleagues.

Being Essential

Research from previous pandemics has described the experiences of women as "invisible" and "inconspicuous" (Harman 2016). This is not the case with COVID-19 in Canada – the press and politicians have highlighted the role of women as frontline responders and those providing the majority of care. Headlines read, "Women Are Leading Canada's Public Health Response to the COVID-19 Coronavirus Outbreak," and Prime Minister Trudeau tweeted, "[W]omen have been at the forefront of our fight against COVID-19. From Dr. Tam … to many other public health officials, scientists, and frontline workers across the country, they've been keeping us all safe and healthy" (Foster 2020) (see figure 1.2).

As the following chapters will demonstrate, being labelled essential can be both empowering and disempowering. On the one hand, being labelled essential confers status and recognition. As Mejia et al. (2021) write, "In the context of the COVID-19 pandemic, occupations previously stigmatized, or categorized as "dirty work," have been deemed essential, followed by a marked shift in societal discourse on the value of these occupations." In most Canadian provinces, essential workers, such as nurses and long-term-care aides, saw wage increases through pandemic pay and related initiatives as a means of recognizing their added value within the pandemic response. However, when such status and recognition are not forthcoming or are not matched by material support, it can also highlight injustice and inequities. For example, Folbre, Gautham, and Smith (2021) demonstrate that, in the United States, essential workers in feminized care sectors (such as those described here) are paid less than essential workers in masculinized sectors (such as in law enforcement, waste services, and transportation).

A nuanced analysis also raises questions about which women are celebrated for what contributions. For example, an analysis of media articles about child care and the pandemic found an overwhelming focus on the experiences of working mothers compared with the role of paid childcare providers (Wallace and Goodyear-Grant 2020). Being essential can also restrict one's ability to leave a job, refuse unsafe work, or demand change, intensifying "the prison of care" (Folbre 2008). This is a particularly concerning restriction during an infectious disease pandemic because essential status also signals increased risk. COVID-19 infections in healthcare workers in Canada are disproportionately high, higher than in many comparable countries, indicating that those in essential roles did indeed risk their safety to provide care (CIHI 2021a). Those on the front lines also face additional, often unrecognized risks, such as the mental-health effects described below. Being essential incurs costs, which must be calculated against the benefits to determine whether the benefits of such a status outweigh these costs.

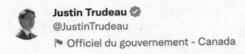

...

Justin Trudeau ✔
@JustinTrudeau
⚐ Officiel du gouvernement - Canada

For the past year, women have been at the forefront of our fight against COVID-19. From Dr. Tam (@CPHO_Canada) to Dr. Nemer (@ChiefSciCan), to many other public health officials, scientists, and front line workers across the country, they've been keeping us all safe and healthy.

2:08 PM · Feb 11, 2021 · Twitter for iPhone

Figure 1.2 Tweet from Prime Minister Justin Trudeau

Not all the professions included in this book are defined as essential according to the Province of British Columbia, where the majority of this research was conducted. The Government of British Columbia defines essential services as "those daily services essential to preserving life, health, public safety and basic societal functioning. They are the services British Columbians come to rely on in their daily lives" (Government of BC 2020). Midwives are not included in this definition and are instead defined as Allied Health, alongside professions such as chiropractic and physiotherapy. Despite this difference, I have included midwives in this research, recognizing that they provide care to 25 per cent of parents and newborns in the province (Stoll and Gallagher 2019). I have also included moms as the essential providers of care to children. Because of necessary limitations, I have focused on key roles related to care work, which includes the health, social assistance, and education sectors.

Mental Health, Moral Distress, and Burnout

COVID-19 has created a mental health crisis in which women are particularly affected. Even before the pandemic, women experienced more barriers to accessing care despite experiencing depression and anxiety twice as often as men (Gadermann et al. 2021). The pandemic led to further disparities in mental health, particularly in women's role in essential paid and unpaid care work. For example, 60 per cent of nurses in BC reported emotional exhaustion, and nearly half (47 per cent) experienced symptoms of post-traumatic stress disorder during the first year of the pandemic (Stelnicki, Carleton, and Reichert 2020). A Canadian Mental Health Association survey found that the number of mothers reporting high anxiety was twice that of the rest of the respondents (CMHA 2020). Reflecting these statistics, the women I spoke to repeatedly described high levels of stress and anxiety alongside experiences of trauma and depression. Consequently, though I did not intend to conduct research on mental health, it became a prominent theme in my conversations with essential workers.

To engage with this theme while drawing on my FPE background, I began with questions about the structural determinants of poor mental health. It is easy to blame the pandemic, which has been stressful for all of us, as the source of all mental health threats. Yet, public policy and interventions determined how the pandemic was experienced and by whom, the types of challenges women on the front lines faced, and the supports available to deal with them. The women who share their experiences here, as will be demonstrated, were rarely suffering because of medical conditions but because of staff shortages and gender norms that increased their responsibilities at work and at home while reducing the support available. Therefore, the corresponding solution might not be primarily medical, such as antidepressants, or even behavioural, such as counselling, but structural.

To unpack the structural determinants of poor mental health during the pandemic, I apply the concept of moral distress. The concept of moral distress – the experience in which one knows the ethically right action to take but is systemically constrained from taking it – was originally developed in the nursing literature in the 1980s and has increasingly been applied to understand the experiences of other healthcare workers, including physicians, those working in long-term care, and social workers (Jameton 1993; Pauly, Varcoe, and Storch 2012). While there are varying conceptualizations and classifications of moral distress, the research converges on the concept of moral distress as occurring when healthcare professionals feel they are being involuntarily complicit in an unethical act but have little power to act differently or change the situation. Constraints that prevent healthcare providers from meeting ethical standards of care may be individual, institutional, or societal. These may come in the form of limited human and healthcare resources (i.e., inadequate time with patients due to staffing shortages); policies and regulations (such as those that restrict patients' access to visitors); tensions between families and staff members/management (e.g., when families demand care that the provider is unwilling or unable to provide); and the isolation of care providers (e.g., being unable to share experiences due to confidentiality protocols) (Pijl-Zieber et al. 2008). The characteristics of moral distress include those inherent in the situation (i.e., that a moral judgment is not acted upon), as well as emotional responses (e.g., guilt, frustration, and feelings of worthlessness) and physiological symptoms (e.g., heart palpitations and diarrhea) (Epstein and Hurst 2017). Experiences of moral distress can lead to heightened levels of stress and burnout and providers leaving the profession. As a result, moral distress not only negatively affects providers' health and well-being but also severely affects health and care systems already struggling with human resource shortages.

There is a growing literature on moral distress during emergencies and crises. Research from healthcare workers during the early part of the HIV/AIDS pandemic and recent Ebola outbreaks often viewed treating patients with communicable diseases as an occupational risk arising from their ethical obligation to provide care. Maunder, writing about the physiological toll of SARS (2002 and 2003), describes a "catastrophe" to the "psychological cost of an infection" due to systems that caused abrupt and discontinuous change (Maunder 2009). Sese, Ahmad, and Rajendram (2020) note that the incompatibility of ethical frameworks in non-pandemic times, focused on patient-centred approaches, and pandemic responses, focused on community-based approaches, can lead to moral distress. They write, "[C]aregivers are now caring for patients in ways that might not have been considered optimal in the context of pre-pandemic ethical frameworks. This shift heightens the potential for moral distress" (Sese, Ahmad, and Rajendram 2020). Examples of COVID-19-related moral distress include not being able to provide high-quality care due to time or resource constraints and not being able to go above and beyond in the type of care provided due to enforced restrictions (Morley et al. 2020).

A number of studies have revealed higher levels of moral distress among women healthcare workers than men (Pinquart and Sörensen 2006). Such differences may reflect the gendered structures of health systems, wherein more women than men fill positions requiring close contact with patients but have less access to decision-making and/or reflect dominant gender norms within which women are expected to seek personal development by caring for others. O'Connell (2015) notes that psychological studies have found that women have higher levels of moral sensitivity, potentially making them more vulnerable to moral distress.

Despite evidence of gendered differences in experiences of moral distress, feminist analysis of those differences is limited, with most research documenting rather than critically analyzing the prevalence of moral distress (Brassolotto et al. 2017; Pauly, Varcoe, and Storch 2012). Yet, moral distress is an organizational problem that frontline workers experience on a personal level, making it particularly suited to a feminist analysis that aims to illuminate the relationship between the public and private realm, and between individual agency and structural power (Pijl-Zieber et al. 2008). In highlighting the contributions of unpaid care to the health and social care sector, feminist analysis suggests that the concept of moral distress can be applied to both unpaid and paid care responsibilities. While the care economy literature has documented the obligation of parents to care for children and the distress that arises when parents are unable to meet the standards of care they deem appropriate, it has not considered these experiences as moral distress. Hossain (2021), in a study of moral distress among physicians, notes that the conflict between the moral obligation to serve and treat patients and the moral obligation to protect one's family/dependents can lead to moral conflict. Beyond pointing out these tensions, little in-depth analysis has been done on whether essential workers experience moral distress in relation to their unpaid and paid care responsibilities and the resulting possibility of multiple experiences of distress. Yet, not only is most health, elder, and child care unpaid and conducted in the home by women, most health and social care workers – being women – fulfill both paid and unpaid care roles. The following chapters therefore identify experiences of moral distress in both paid and unpaid care work.

Power

Much of the research on women and COVID-19 describes the material effects of COVID-19 – the lost jobs and increased care work – with some starting to document the mental health effects, all key themes included in this book. Less discussed is how the pandemic has affected women's power to effect change, how women have exercised power within it, and to what effect. Yet the concept of power is at the heart of

feminist research and analysis, which has advanced recognition of the
need to critically unpack power relations within the formal workforce
and the home (McPhail 2003). The limited research on women and
power in the context of COVID-19 focuses on how many women are
represented in decision-making. For example, one early assessment
found that 85 per cent of 115 COVID-19 task forces from eighty-seven
countries consisted primarily of men (van Daalen et al. 2020). The
organization Women in Global Health has highlighted that only
20 per cent of the WHO Emergency Committee on COVID-19 are
women (WGH 2020). Canada is an outlier when it comes to the gender
composition of COVID-19 leadership. Not only is the federal chief
public health officer a woman of Asian descent, but the majority of
provincial health officers at the time of the outbreak were also women.
The provincial health officer in British Columbia, Dr Bonnie Henry,
has been particularly celebrated for her leadership, and is often
described using terms associated with femininity, such as "comforting"
(Porter 2020). While perceptions of Dr Henry's policies have become
more diverse as the pandemic has continued, she has retained her position as a powerful leader of the response.

However, the gender composition of leadership is just one metric
of power, and a weak one at that. The focus on representation
equates the presence of women with equity, assuming that these
women will advance equity agendas and will have the power to do
so. As Wenham and Herten-Crabb (2021) write, "In exalting wom-
en's executive leadership as the signpost for equality, we inculcate
the idea that individual women can independently overcome patriarchal structures (i.e., 'if they only try hard enough') and obscure
the plight of millions of women who do not benefit from such a
position." The participation of (or consultation with) women does
not guarantee that action will be taken to address gender inequities
and can be limited by many factors: formal and informal rules,
institutional cultures, and women's disproportionate share of unpaid
care work, which reduces the time they have available to participate
(Davies et al. 2019). The increase in women's unpaid care work and
the emotional labour demanded by the pandemic response is a particular threat to women's ability to participate in decision-making
and leadership.

Intersectional feminism recognizes that power is multifaceted
because of intersecting structures of privilege and oppression.
D'Ignazio and Klein define power as:

[t]he current configuration of structural privilege and
structural oppression, in which some groups experience
unearned advantages – because various systems have been
designed by people like them and work for people them – and
other groups experience systematic disadvantages – because
those same systems were not designed by them or with people
like them in mind. (2020, 4)

These structures are often taken for granted, with the inequities they
generate either ignored or accepted. As a result, examining power
means naming and explaining the forces of oppression that are "so
baked into our daily lives that we often ignore them" (D'Ignazio and
Klein 2020, 4).

In this book, questions of power emerge in how essential women
workers are positioned within the hierarchies of the health and
education systems and the broader society and community. The book
explores who has a voice and can effect change in decision-making
and who cannot, and why, as well as who feels their concerns are
heard and responded to, and who does not. These questions revolve
around the inequities that result in women not having the resources
(including time) to participate in leadership and challenge gender
norms. For example, lack of access to child care reflects institutional
priorities that restrict women's career and income-related opportunities, which in turn interact with gender norms that are reflected
in wage gaps to force women to give up paid work when child care
cannot be found. Questions also emerge around safety and security
and how the COVID-19 response decreased both for many women.
This broad definition of power aims to illustrate the multiple
configurations that structure power over women during times
of crisis.

Structures of power are, of course, not absolute. Women in Canada
and around the world continue to challenge them, having achieved,
among other efforts, recent gains in equal pay legislation, investments
in child care, and shifting gender norms. Because the revolution for
gender equality remains a work in progress, documenting acts of
empowerment and resistance to the current structures of inequity is
as important, if not more important, than documenting continued
expressions of patriarchy (Tallis 2012). Therefore, this book analyzes
both the power structures that shaped women's experiences of the
pandemic and their efforts to transform them.

CONCLUSION

I began this book from a place of hope. Inspired by the experiences of the women who staffed the front lines of the response, I wanted to share their stories so that their sacrifices and contributions would be recognized. I believed, and I still do, that we can learn a great deal from these experiences that can enable us to both reflect on and heal from the COVID-19 pandemic and be better prepared for future health crises. Over the past two years of pandemic waves, I have also come to see this book as an act of resistance. Many people's opposition to public health measures and the failure to address the ongoing secondary effects placed disproportionately on women demand a response. This book is my retort to calls to return to "normal," recognizing that normal is not good enough and if that's all we did would continue to set up our health, education, and care sectors to be just as vulnerable to crisis as the pandemic has proven they already were. To create a more resilient future, we must first centre the empowerment and well-being of those we all depend on when we are at our most vulnerable – women who care.

2

The Underdogs

Long-Term-Care Staff

I feel like this is a problem that belongs to everyone in our society,
like the pandemic is shining a light on all aspects of how we organize care,
how we value our elders, and how we value the work of those who serve
our elders. We're the underdogs in the health system.

Long-term-care aide

There is a scene in the movie *Gallipoli* where young Australian men
are sent over the trench to certain death. It is a compelling and clear
depiction of the futility of war, of how the ignorance and hubris
of those in power put those young men in an impossible situation.
The main character, played by a young Mel Gibson, is tasked with
running a message that could stop his best friend from being sent
over the top, and he, a former athlete, runs with all his might but
doesn't make it in time. It doesn't end well. I often thought of both
scenes, the soldiers going over the top to a battle they could not win
and the young runner going all out in the hope of saving a life, when
I was reading the transcripts from those working in long-term care
(LTC) during COVID-19.

The media reported the first COVID-19 death on 9 March 2020 in an
LTC facility in BC (Seyd 2020). LTC facilities, homes where seniors
who are unable to care for themselves live with the support of care
aides and others, quickly became the epicentre of the COVID-19 pandemic in Canada, with 55 per cent of all deaths between March 2020
and March 2022 occurring in LTC (CIHI 2021b). Canada subsequently

earned the dubious distinction of having the highest proportion of LTC COVID-19 deaths in any OECD country. And care aides in LTC were the most likely of all health professionals to contract COVID-19 (CIHI 2021a). In addition to the immediate health risk of COVID-19 infection, those working in LTC faced increased workloads alongside overwhelming trauma and grief.

Over 90 per cent of those working in LTC identify as women. Among OECD countries, Canada spends 30 per cent less than the average on LTC, despite seniors' advocates, among others, repeatedly calling for increased public investment in the sector as well as national standards (Estabrooks et al. 2020). In BC, the sector includes a mix of publicly funded facilities operated by health authorities (33 per cent), for-profit companies (35 per cent), and not-for-profit societies (32 per cent) contracted by the health authorities. A 2020 report found that the for-profit sector generated twelve times more profit/surplus than the non-profit sector, but spent 24 per cent less on direct care per resident (Office of the Seniors Advocate 2020).

Variation in the sector has resulted in a wide range of work environments, though staffing shortages and high rates of burnout are common across facilities, with 60 per cent of operators experiencing staffing shortages in 2017 (SafeCare BC 2017). Pre-COVID-19, workers were often subjected to exhausting and unpredictable workloads, including inconsistently assigned work hours, with over 30 per cent working more than one job (Duan et al. 2020). In 2019, those working in LTC reported declining emotional well-being and fear of taking sick leave because of the risk of losing employment (Office of the Seniors Advocate 2020).

Following the initial COVID-19 outbreaks in LTC facilities, it became apparent that having workers in part-time positions at multiple facilities was unsafe. After consulting with unions and employers, the BC government instituted a single-site order, which meant that each employee could only work at one facility. This was accompanied by a minimum pay floor of $20 per hour for care aides (previously, some had been making less than $12 per hour) and an agreement that workers would not earn overtime pay (because employers argued the single-site order made overtime a necessity and they could not afford the extra cost) (Duan et al. 2020). Meanwhile, because visitors and volunteers were no longer allowed inside the facilities, staff had to take on additional care work. National media reports depicted dire conditions inside locked-down care facilities, including residents going without meals, baths, and medical care (Cecco 2020). Most of this coverage focused on the experiences of residents, not staff, who were either left out of the story or indirectly blamed for residents' poor care.

This chapter includes perspectives from a wide range of women working in the LTC sector during the first year of the pandemic. The focus group participants (23) and interviewees (4) ranged from those working in housekeeping and food service to recreational assistants and care aides, to managers and unit clerks. Women also came from a variety of facility types, including public, for-profit, and non-profit. The range of perspectives is unique in that it includes those from a variety of roles and with differing responsibilities, generating a complex picture of the conditions within the sector. This chapter aims to highlight these women's contributions and expose the cracks within the system that often made it impossible for them to do their jobs when and where they were most needed.

THE QUADRUPLE BURDEN

The combination of a chronically understaffed sector and the single-site order, which increased staffing challenges and the need for staff exposed or symptomatic to isolate, on top of pandemic protocols creating new tasks, exponentially increased the workload of all those working in LTC. A recreation support worker explained:

> A lot of the exhausting part in our work is just being short-staffed with the single-site order. [I]t really affected us; all departments are short-staffed. In my department, which is recreation, normally we have six, we're down to two. And plus, the added work that's been given to us with COVID, you know, the visits, and the Zoom and the phone calls and all that, on top of our regular work, trying to keep the residents busy, it's exhausting. I come home and I'm done.

Efforts to increase staffing were inhibited by low pay and poor working conditions. One custodial worker explained: "They doubled the amount of staff that we have since COVID, and it's a rotating door. Every day I go to work, there's two or three new people. But we never seem to go over one hundred people, so we must be losing two or three a day … we're always short staffed, we always have positions in our area that aren't filled." A care aide noted, "[T]here's nobody coming to work, because we can't pay them enough to show up." Another housekeeper noted, "[T]hey're having a very hard time keeping people. Just the last day, they were missing a housekeeper. She showed up and just said, I'm out of here after one day. And it's just, like, rotating door of staff, nobody's trained, and just everybody's so angry, like, really angry, because all this more workload and we're just getting paid such crappy wages."

While the provincial government instituted changes to ensure that all employees in the sector had full-time work and instituted a $20 salary floor (barely equal to a living wage in the Lower Mainland of BC), many found that the compensation still did not correspond to their workload. Workers were not paid extra for overtime yet felt compelled to work overtime due to the high need and lack of staff. One care aide described, "Working sixteen hours and twenty-four hours sometimes because nobody wants to come in … Because working overtime, there's no pay for overtime. That's what we experienced at work." A manager noted that her staff had worked two and a half times more overtime than the same month the previous year.

These shortages affected patient care, with workers having to make calculations about what services to cut.

> There's plenty days where we're working, even just short staffed, there's been plenty of nights where I've been doing one to twenty-two ratios. So, it's heavy, it's a lot of work, it's a lot on a person. There's a lot of, not shortcuts but things like who can you keep in bed for dinner, who can you put in pajamas? I think the biggest thing that we end up cutting out first, for example, their baths.

In 2019, the BC Care Providers Association recommended that each resident receive at least 3.36 hours of direct care a day. During staffing shortages, one care aide might be responsible for the care of twenty-two residents, which equals seventy-four hours of care work per day – an impossible equation. Consequently, care providers had to skip necessities, which affected resident care:

> But there is multiple times where people are missing their baths for four-plus weeks. When it gets to that point, and it's been a month and that's on the residency, you feel bad because there are people, and this is their homes and their lives potentially,

right. And they're not getting the care that they need and so how I mean it always ends up coming back on us is we have to eventually just have to stop and find the energy or find the time – it eventually just catches up to us. The work just doesn't disappear, we just don't do it for that day.

Despite already being overworked, the women working in LTC took on additional tasks to mitigate residents' isolation during lockdown. Residents' family members, desperate for connection, reached out to those working in LTC via social media and other means, asking for information about their family members and support so they could communicate with them. Recognizing the urgent need for connection, many women used their personal phones and their own time to connect residents to family members. A recreation assistant explained:

When COVID hit, all of our families were locked down, locked away and all our volunteers, all of the support people that generally just make a long-term-care facility a community, were not able to come in. And so, we picked up these things to try and connect. We picked up assisting care aides with some care, we picked up trying to keep our families in touch with residents, through Skype or FaceTime. There were all these tiny little duties that we had that didn't ever seem very big. But when you look at them sort of in retrospect, I look at the whole package, and it was just exhausting. Just the amount of extra work we had was just almost on every level, was really exhausting.

Similarly, a care aide noted:

I became friends with a lot of family members on Facebook and, because they weren't allowed in the building, they would message me and say, "OK, can you be in Dad's room at such and such a time? Do you have time?" And I go, "Yeah, yeah." And I would go in the room so that they could video chat with their loved one. So, between doing that and then having to get all my work done that same day, I'd get like twenty messages a day.

Others took on additional tasks to support residents' well-being. One housekeeper described becoming "the Shaw technician when Shaw couldn't come in." She set up all the televisions and got the Shaw package working because "I believe that these people should have television when they're stuck in a room, right? So, I took that role on, and I was very happy to do that."

In addition to connecting residents with family, workers felt the need to provide the in-person connection that was missing. A recreational assistant explained:

> You find that you had to be more so their confidante and their only real social contact that they were having during that time was one of us coming in three times a day for five or twenty minutes, however long their care needs were. And those often ended up getting stretched out because they did need that contact and you're only one person, you can only do so much. There's where your workload was greatly increased.

Such emotional labour increased care aides' sense of purpose and job satisfaction, with many women expressing gratitude that they had meaningful work during the pandemic. One care aide reflected, "I am thankful for my job every day. That I can honestly say, that when my feet hit the floor, thank you that this is the reason my feet hit the floor at five o'clock in the morning, you know, to go and be with the residents and support them because they deserve it."

Many women working in long-term care also had care responsibilities at home, which were affected by their increased professional workload. Women described "almost sleeping at work" and never being able to take time off due to a lack of replacement staff. A care aide with young children noted, "I'm you know, a little bit more exhausted when I come home, so I'm not, you know, the same nurturing type person that I know that I have been in the past with my family." Another described, "You give, give, give all day and you do your best to give all day and then you go home depleted, but you still have to give at home. Because you go home and you're still a mom, and you still have to cook, and shop, and clean and all of that stuff and try to be the best you can be there." Increased demands at work left less energy and time to meet needs that were just as pressing at home.

Respondents struggled with the balance of providing care to extended family and reducing the risk of exposure for themselves, their families, and the residents for whom they cared. At times, the decision to reduce contact with family members led to conflict. One care aide explained that her parents were getting mad at me for not letting them see their grandkids and I'm like, I work at a care home and my father-in-law is elderly and he has cancer and stuff, and so I will not put anyone I care about at risk. I really care about the residents I work with, and they weren't understanding of that, they took it really personally. And so that was really hard because I had to stand my ground.

Another mother noted that her decision to maintain contact with grandparents who provided child care, but not other family members, led to conflict: "We have to choose our bubble based on who's caring for our children, and it's hard because you don't choose based on who you love the most, you choose on what's practical in your life. And yeah, so that's been really challenging. Trying to deal with our own well-being and then kind of trying to field other people's well-being when you don't have the capacity, right." The constant trade-offs between risk and care responsibilities increased women's emotional labour.

Such choices became even more difficult when women were providing essential care to older adults both at work and at home. A facility manager summarized the conflict between the first and second shift through an example from one of the care aides in her facility:

Grandma wants to go into assisted living, but mom just died so now granddaughter has to take care of her. The granddaughter is a fulltime employee of mine, she's stressed out, she's in my office in tears 90 per cent of the time because she can't get her grandma a place because of COVID. Grandma's on the island, she can't even go see her. If she does, she's bending the rules. So, she moves Grandma in to live with her. Now she's got Grandma in her house with her two teenage boys, with her husband, with her dog, like that's one tiny example. Yet, she still comes to work every day and she faces work, and she makes a better life for people.

In some cases, it was impossible for women to fulfill both care responsibilities. One care aide left her job because she was the sole care provider to an elderly mother. She described "struggling with having made that choice because it feels like I'm letting my co-workers down. Because I had to make that decision to protect myself and protect my mom." Another described "getting pulled in those two directions of, I want to be there for my co-workers, but I need to protect my family."

These fears were well-founded, because LTC care aides had the highest rate of COVID infection of all healthcare workers in Canada (CIHI 2021a), and many had witnessed instances of people bringing COVID home from outbreaks and passing it on to their family members or vice versa. Knowing this risk affected respondents' own well-being. "I feel I've – I was worried that I was going to be the one to take it into work. I walked around, as we all have, with so much angst that every day would be tears and hoping that I didn't have it and I wanted to not be around my family, because I didn't want them to give me something and me take it into work." A representative from an organization of care aides noted that a member survey showed that care aides' biggest fear was not getting COVID-19 themselves but passing it on to a resident.

While concern for others caused high levels of anxiety and necessitated difficult decisions, women also recognized that they generated strength through the care roles that they applied at work. A care aide explained, "[W]e're nurturers, we're moms and we nurture at work, this is who we are no matter what." Another said, "I think thankfully a lot of us care aides have got that mom skin, where it just, we still just pick up and keep going no matter what. I mean I don't know what we would do if we had enough staff. I think a lot of the care aides would stand around and stare at each other like what is this? Free time, what?"

BEING ESSENTIAL

Pre-COVID-19, the work of care aides in LTC was not celebrated as an essential service; in fact, often, the opposite was true. Badone (2021) argues that both LTC workers and residents have been marginalized in Canada by societal attitudes toward aging, disability, and death. A care aide described how LTC was thought of, if it was thought of at all, as "yucky smelly places where people go to die." She went on to describe how this dismissal limited the ability of the sector to respond to the pandemic: "You know, nobody even wants to work here because it's not glamorous work. Like that's the stigma we've attached to long-term care, and we saw that reflected in some ways in the pandemic itself." An LTC manager similarly felt that stigma toward the sector reflected societal attitudes toward aging and death, saying, "You know, the problems that we saw in the pandemic are really the product of ageism that's inherent in our society, and how we organize our systems of care." Relegated to the periphery of health systems as primarily contracted-out care services, LTCs were "under-resourced, underfunded and under-appreciated." A care aide noted that this difference persisted within the pandemic despite LTC being the site of most outbreaks:

> But what was really interesting to me is, we were getting the six o'clock cheer for hospital workers whose – you know in the ICU, you're looking at 52 per cent bed capacity. Whereas, at the same time, we had care homes dealing with these significant outbreaks. And so, you know that to me just pulls out a nice little example of our general attention to this sector. Typically, we'll idolize those who work in acute care, and we kind of forget that long-term care exists ... And I feel like that's indicative of our general approach to long-term care. It's sort of out of sight, out of mind, we don't like to talk about it ... it's always been the underdog. It's always been the under-resourced, underfunded stepchild, if you will, of the healthcare sector.

The LTC sector's lack of structural integration into the broader public health sector combined with cultural norms about elder care to leave residents and workers vulnerable to the pandemic.

Those working in LTC quickly went from being largely invisible, in terms of public and political recognition, to being in the spotlight due to media coverage of outbreaks. While workers appreciated the recognition as essential workers and its related perks of free food and gifts during the initial months of the pandemic, they were also stigmatized and blamed, particularly as the media portrayed images of neglect within the LTC sector. A care aide noted, "A part that really bothered me is the media with, you know, saying that these residents are put in their rooms, they don't have any love, they don't get to see their family, and I believe our facility bends over backwards to have outdoor visits, patio visits. It's just that part is very frustrating for me." The women felt that the time and sacrifices they were making to ensure care for residents, including working long hours, which resulted in less time with their own families, were unacknowledged, and instead, they were judged on the basis of the worst examples, caused by policies they had no control over. A manager reflected on the hurt caused by the media coverage and public perceptions, saying,

It hurts when people – like the judgment again, I'm just so tired
of people judging. You get judged because you put people in
long-term care, so of course you just tie them to a chair and,
you know, feed them slop and ignore them and lock them in
a room. Apparently, that's what we do. And it would be nice –
if you could meet half of my staff, like the females, the ones that
were in tears today because – like we lost one of our residents
who we loved.

Women felt that the images of LTC portrayed in the media and the
concerns being voiced in public did not reflect their experiences of
caring deeply for the residents.

Those working in housekeeping and food service felt that they were
not afforded the same "essential" worker status as others, despite the
importance of their work and the risk they assumed in doing it. One
housekeeper described how,

being a housekeeper in a long-term-care home, you're responsible
to make sure that everything is clean. Because if the virus got
into where you're working, I always assume that the first person
they're going to look at is the housekeeper. So, you get tired,
because you got to make sure you wipe everything down three
or four times and then ... you always get paranoid with this
virus being out there. One, I don't want to bring it home to my
loved ones, and, two, to even bring it into the care home and
give it to a senior. I think that would just kill me, because of the
big responsibility ... I can't breathe at all, being at work and at
the same time running around, making sure the virus doesn't
come through that front door.

Despite being responsible for cleanliness, many housekeepers were
not provided with the same standard of PPE (personal protective
equipment) as care aides or nurses. One described being denied gloves
and hand sanitizer and told to wash her hands instead: "Can you
imagine going in and out of rooms? That's what we were using,
soap and water. Which is great, but when you're going into another
room, and you don't have your gloves and you're still wearing
the same mask that you came out of a COVID-positive room." One
worker described nurses being directed to wear N95 masks when
caring for COVID-positive residents, but not the custodial and food

service workers, who were cleaning the same residents' rooms and providing food to them, who were told they didn't need one. In many facilities, doctors, nurses, and care aides were vaccinated before the housekeepers and food service staff, further symbolizing a hierarchy showing whose health and whose safety mattered most. One member of the food service staff described receiving her first dose at the same time as residents' family members, noting, "We're just treated so differently. I don't know. Like I said, like we're the bottom of the shoe."

Housekeepers noted that management in some facilities pushed for workers to come to work even when they were sick and that those on probation were fired for taking time off due to sickness. A housekeeper explained,

> They just say "Oh you're sick? You're still coming to work," that's what we get. We go to work sick … they're actually firing people that aren't coming to work because they're sick. If they're on probation, like, if they're just hired, if they miss three days, they're gone … But that's OK, because we're just housekeepers, like, this is how we're treated. And it got really good there for a bit, everybody was cheering our names, and now it's back to, we're shit on the bottom of the shoe again. It's really sad.

Notably, a report by the Office of the Seniors Advocate of BC (2021) found that sites that provided fewer sick days were more likely to experience larger COVID-19 outbreaks.

Most women felt their contributions to the COVID-19 response were unseen: "I ended up working thirteen days straight and almost a hundred and five hours in the first two weeks of outbreak. And when I brought it up to management about kind of needing the support, I was kind of told, 'I work that much, I worked a hundred hours as well.' And that kind of set me into the point where it's like you don't care about the staff." Another noted, "I was flabbergasted that not once in the last year has our manager kind of gathered us together and said like, 'Well done, team' or 'I see how hard you're working' or anything. That would kind of just really acknowledge how hard we were working and how complex it was." Others repeated how far simple recognition could go: "I just feel like they needed to – and even if it's just say thanks and just the words. We realize how hard you guys are working … that alone [would] probably bring out whatever it is by like 20 per cent if we just heard those words come out on a

person-to-person basis." Another woman described how powerful
shows of appreciation can be: "[O]ur employer sort of set up an email
system so that all of the friends and family could write and show their
appreciation to the staff. And that [was] actually quite lovely, so we
had people that would, you know, like send encouragement to everybody or thank everybody."

MENTAL HEALTH,
MORAL DISTRESS, AND BURNOUT

Before COVID-19, longitudinal research documented declining mental health among LTC care aides, a trend worsened by COVID-19
(Havaei et al. 2022). Women working in long-term care described
multiple incidents of moral distress when they were unable to meet
the care needs of residents due to staff shortages. One care aide
explained, "It doesn't feel good to leave people without having a bath
for four weeks. It doesn't feel good to not put that lipstick on that
one lady who it just brightens up her whole day." Another reflected,
"It's really scary to think that we're asked to do our jobs in such an
environment where we can't. We can't do what we want to do and
how we want to do it." Another explained that the constant need to
cut corners weighed on her: "Well you can leave the residents up and
the night shift can put them to bed or whatever. But just for me
personally, having done this job for so long, I didn't feel very good
going home ... My mental health took a big toll." The women
explained that their inability to provide quality care led to burnout,
"and you kind of are reduced to providing a lesser quality of care and
that does not feel good. Right you don't go away feeling proud
and feeling, oh well I can't wait to go back tomorrow ... I've seen
more people feeling more jaded. I've seen cares and nurses, the regular
ones who are working becoming more burnt out because they're
having to carry that burden."

Care aides also experienced moral distress in response to the loneli-
ness of residents who were unable to receive visitors: "I'm on the floor
dealing with people who are upset and lonely and sad because they
don't have husbands, or spouses, or family coming to see them ...
I think the frustrating thing is just sometimes not being able to help
somebody who's inconsolable because they're crying, missing a spouse,
or just being exhausted, and you know that part of it I think I find
very frustrating." Participants felt helpless having to impose public

health measures they recognized as causing harm. A manager of an LTC facility noted, "The residents were sad that they couldn't see their families, the families were upset that they couldn't see their loved ones. And I had no control over any of it. I just didn't have the solutions for them." The isolation of residents created a layering of moral dilemmas – care providers felt they should increase the comfort they provided but remained restricted from doing so.

Many respondents described themselves as paranoid about avoiding COVID-19 infection, not out of fear for themselves but (as described above) for those they provided care to. Some workers described their compulsion to repeatedly clean both their worksite and their home: "It's always in the front of your mind, right, not in the back of your mind, but it's always in the front, right? It's like 'OK, well did I wash my hands,' you know, or my mask is once again falling off my nose, and so I'm fixing it, and then they're like 'Well now you've contaminated your mask.'" Another respondent said,

> My brain is constantly, "OK, did I do this at work? Oh, no, what if I didn't do that?" My whole demeanour has changed, like, me, personally. When somebody comes into my house – because you're allowed so many now – that I have hand sanitizer at my front door. "Can you sanitize before you come in?" And I have teenage kids, that when they come in the door I'm, like, "Hand sanitize and then go to the kitchen." ... They're like, "Relax." I'm like, "No." I'm over – I don't want to say over paranoid, but I feel like I am over paranoid now.

The women felt the need to "hold yourself up with a higher standard" and related this to their gendered role as care providers: "First of all I am a mother of four and I have a grandchild too. When you are a mother, you want to protect your whole household, and that goes with your patients, your work as well." Such feelings of responsibility combined with fear of infection increased their anxiety, or what workers described as paranoia.

Those working in LTC must regularly grapple with grief, a challenge even during non-pandemic times due to conflicting feelings of care for residents alongside recognition of the nature of LTC, which is ultimately end-of-life care. COVID-19 not only added to incidents of grief but complicated them, further increasing premature and unpredictable deaths. One manager noted, "With the second wave of the pandemic, having significant deaths and mortality in long-term-care settings has been profound. And it's challenging for people who work in long-term care in general because we grapple with this question of the right to grieve, and do I have the right to mourn this person's passing, because they were dear and close to me but they're not my family." That grief extended to all those working in contact with residents.

> We were losing residents that you become very close with. Even though I'm a housecleaner. We were really hit hard. You become part of their family. Even when they do pass – before COVID-19 hit you were going to these residents' funerals. Because you're part of them. And they say you're not supposed to be part of them, you've got to separate. How can you? You work day in and day out with these people, that I look at every one of them either as my parent or my grandparent. I hold a very, very big spot in my heart for all of them.

A care aide who experienced an outbreak in an LTC facility noted that the increase in deaths caused her to fall into a depression: "When I went off work, I would come home and I'm like people are dying, there's nothing I can do about it. I became obsessed with death. I couldn't eat, I couldn't sleep … I'm like, 'People are dying I've got to do something.' But there's nothing I can do."

Dealing with these challenges every day, many women spoke of feeling isolated. One said, "Just working in a care facility, the residents aren't getting their families coming in … And I find when I am outside of work, I don't see many people either. I find both on my job and in my personal life I just feel very alone and isolated and it's not OK." Most women noted that they had greatly reduced contact with friends and family to mitigate the risk of transmission. One woman noted, "I have really been struggling with, I haven't seen my granddaughter in a while. My mom, she's ill. So, I stay away from her because she is compromised. I've noticed I don't sleep really well." The inability to connect with social networks disables coping mechanisms and emotional supports, restricting opportunities for recreation and connecting with those outside the sector: "But it's been very isolating. We haven't seen friends. I'm just too scared. And my friends are still partying with other people who are not in their bubble." Confidentiality protocols further restricted opportunities to share with those outside the sector.

What I found extra challenging is, we're bound by confidentiality. We go to work, whatever happens at work, we can't talk about it. So, you get – and because all of us, housekeeping, food services, everybody involved, is overworked, we're doing twelve-hour days, you might be able to catch three minutes with a coworker going, "Oh, my God, like, are you losing it today?" "Heck yeah." And then, you come home, and you can't talk about it. You can't talk about what's going on at work.

The inability to speak about the challenges at work with friends and family meant that women often felt they had to deal with stress and anxiety on their own.

LTC facilities provided mental health support through virtual and tele-peer support programs, but many noted little uptake. A manager commented, "I would like to force people to receive education on self-care and on coping skills. Because we never force them, we always just make it available and the people that utilize it are few and far between." Previous research on worker well-being in LTC similarly found that most workers did not access employee assistance programs, often not trusting them to be confidential, finding virtual support unhelpful, or being deterred by the application process (Goldberg et al. 2022). The women further noted that their heavy workloads prevented them from accessing mental wellness supports, explaining that calling a counsellor would not address the sources of their distress, such as being unable to provide quality care due to their workload, as described above.

A number of women noted that they would have appreciated opportunities for in-person peer mental health support:

I would have liked to have seen more mental support, like group chat … As a whole, we kind of weren't given the opportunity to meet up with managers and have a huddle. It was kind of we were flying by the seats of our pants. For the first six months literally, they didn't ask us how we were. It was unbelievable. So, the mental support from our managers, I would've liked to have seen more of.

Previous research with care aides found that talking to peers helped alleviate moral distress but that such support was constrained by heavy workloads and organizational norms (Brassolotto et al. 2017). In the context of COVID-19, physical distancing exacerbated barriers to this coping mechanism because workers couldn't gather in break rooms or meet after work for a chat. However, a few facilities did take steps to foster peer support, which was highly appreciated:

> We really as a team, we really try to just grab ten minutes at the very end of the day so we can decompress, because of the confidentiality and all that kind of stuff, you just really needed to talk it out and we can't talk it out with our families. And some of what goes on in long-term care is just too hard to talk about to someone that doesn't work there. It was nice to just kind of, just have that decompress for ten minutes before we went home. We really valued that. We really worked hard to make that happen.

Others noted that COVID-19 workshops that were meant to be skill-building often turned into impromptu peer support events, and that these opportunities were far more valuable than any coping skills.

POWER

Many women working in LTC face daily threats to their personal security. Before COVID-19, the LTC sector had one of the highest rates of workplace injuries and claims (McCloskey, Donovan, and Donovan 2017). The claims were the result of the physical nature of the work, which required lifting and moving residents and the risk of violence from residents. A care aide described how her workplace once put up a calendar and asked workers to put a red dot for every day they were physically or verbally attacked by a resident, "And that calendar was red for the whole month, but did that change anything? No ... I mean who hasn't been spat on, kicked, punched, told that they were many names throughout their shift? And it's a norm." Another explained:

> Well residents, they come into the workplace because they have Parkinson's, they have other disabilities that make them lash out. It makes them swear, it makes them kick, it makes them punch, it makes them – a lot of it is not controlled and a lot of it is what it is, that is their disease. It's not them, it's their disease, and you have to keep reminding yourself that. But when you're short-staffed and you're trying to dress a person that's a puncher or kicker or whatever, it's violence in the workplace.

Pre-COVID-19, residents' distress could be mitigated by support from family members and volunteers who helped with basic care tasks, offered emotional support, and provided recreational opportunities. COVID-19-related lockdowns prevented both family members and volunteers from visiting, not only isolating residents, but also increasing their emotional distress and therefore likelihood to be violent toward care workers.

This violence was often accompanied by racism, with incidents of racism increasing during the pandemic. A survey conducted during the first year of the pandemic found that visible minority groups were three times more likely than the rest of the population to have experienced an increase in race-based harassment or attacks, with Asian respondents feeling the most at risk (Shore 2020). In July 2021, more than half of Asian Canadians surveyed said they had suffered discrimination over the past year. In Vancouver, anti-Asian hate crimes increased 717 per cent during the first year of the COVID-19 pandemic (Statistics Canada 2020b). Women of Asian descent working in LTC reported being told to "go back to China" and having residents refuse their care. One LTC care aide reflected that while racism and violence from residents had occurred before the pandemic, it had since increased: "What I see is the pandemic just increased frequency of the experiences or the way that people like show us in their attitude, behaviours, or the weight of the hatred that they are showing has increased with the pandemic. But it was there before that too, it just levelled up." Racism also came from colleagues and supervisors. Indigenous women and those from racial minorities spoke of being made to feel that they were more likely to bring COVID-19 into facilities. Others reported being told not to speak their first language during breaks, which limited their access to peer support to deal with stress and anxiety. In addition to this outright racism, focus group participants and interviewees noted systemic discrimination. For example, in most LTC facilities, COVID-19 information was only provided in English, despite English not being the first language for over 70 per cent of those working in LTC (Lightman 2021).

Within this context, many LTC workers felt that their resources or opportunities to inform decision-makers of the challenges they faced were limited. Most described a top-down organizational structure that emphasized obeying protocols, leaving little room for them to consult or be consulted or participate in decision-making. While recognizing the need for defined public health measures, the women described feeling that protocols were imposed without providing them opportunities for input. A manager noted,

> So, the Ministry of Health, which has put in I think a sincere effort to engage, but I also think a lot of decisions were made and implemented very quickly, with little opportunity for wider engagement in the sector, and, in particular, the people doing the actual work ... I think that's one of the major challenges is, we had that command-and-control centre structure, where it was like this is the order and then do it. And when it hit the floor, it was like, wait, it's not working. And here's why it's not working. But that feedback didn't have a good loop.

Many noted that the only time they interacted with those making decisions was during inspections, when representatives from the health authorities would visit the facilities to ensure they were following protocols: "[T]hey seemed to funnel a lot of regulations. We heard a lot about what we couldn't do and the regulations, but the only time we got somebody in from sort of higher up in health authority was when we were being inspected to see if we were following all the protocols." During such visits, LTC facility staff felt as if they were being judged or graded as opposed to being asked for input or how they might be better supported.

Those working in direct contact with residents felt that protocols were implemented through a punitive approach that enforced the power of the employer and health authority over the care providers. One described her manager standing with a clipboard and timer, monitoring how long each person spent washing their hands. Another explained, "[W]e've got thermometers everywhere, and we've got to log all this stuff and God help you if you're caught doing anything different than this new policy and procedure that was just brought in ten minutes ago, right?" Punitive approaches added to the stress workers were already dealing with: "Instead of being like, you guys did great and keep it up, we actually got an email sent to us saying, 'If you don't wear your PPE proper, you will be dismissed ... If you don't do this, you will get punished.' We weren't supported, we were actually put in fear mode of we have to do everything proper of X, Y and Z, otherwise we'll get in trouble." Such pressure was particularly acute when care providers were then responsible for ensuring that residents followed protocols, being forced to further enforce the chain of command. A recreational assistant explained, "Protocols say we have to be six feet apart and everyone has dementia and they're lonely. And you see people come up to each other and hold hands, then it's our job to break them apart and make sure that they're six feet apart or we're going to get in trouble. I just thought that was just so heartless."

Many women noted that protocols were dictated by those distanced from the reality of daily care work during a pandemic. Senior management often worked from home or a secluded office to maintain physical distancing, which meant they did not witness the effects of the policies they were implementing. Care aides described feeling that this positioning created an unnecessary conflict wherein they tried to explain why a policy was not working or was harmful, while managers demanded enforcement: "I felt like almost at times we became the enemy. And so, it felt like trust somehow got broken between us and management." This top-down approach was particularly frustrating when protocols were questionable. One respondent noted that residents were not allowed to read the newspaper until two days after it arrived out of a fear of surface contamination, but visitors could drop off gifts that were provided right away. At times, care providers found ways around the regulations they felt were unnecessary. For example, when they were told they could not put up a Christmas tree, they set one up on the balcony.

Despite the abundance of protocols, many care aides, housekeepers, and others did not, at least during the initial phase of the pandemic, have the information they needed to feel empowered to keep themselves safe. Many described not knowing what they were walking into at their job sites. One woman described an early outbreak in her facility:

When the outbreak first happened, there was no communication about what floor had it or where it was affected. It was kind of by word of mouth, like it was an accident, someone found a paper. That was like an accident that someone found. And then it ended up being – people were showing up to work when there was an outbreak, but they only had a notice on the board once you signed in so you're already kind of in the environment ... because they didn't want to scare people, but by doing that we lost trust in our management team because they weren't open ... We found out that someone was sent to the hospital and they were positive. Any staff that were on that shift knew because they spoke about it, but management decided not to let people know outside of the staffing.

Lack of risk communication affected trust between workers and management. Another care aide noted, "Lack of communication is a big one. When the lockdown first happened, they just changed all the codes on all the doors and came around and took all of our fobs away ... No communication at all. And yeah, when rules changed, they just were changed. There was no – and there was no listening to us or answering questions. It was really frustrating. And I didn't feel supported, I don't think anyone did, honestly." Other women noted that their management did send out information, but in long emails that they did not have time to read and that were not accessible for those with lower English literacy levels. Those working in housekeeping felt they were "the last to know" despite the fact that they also had close contact with residents:

> We don't get told what we're cleaning. And sometimes I'll get
> a call about, I don't want to be gross here, but random feces, you
> don't even know who it came out of. And you'll get calls for that
> and you're like, "Well, now I got to PPE because I have no idea
> what I'm cleaning up here." Like, we don't get told a lot of stuff,
> and it puts us in an unsafe situation, especially if we're not trained
> properly. I actually had to stop a man who didn't speak English
> well, he was going in to clean a COVID-19 room and I was
> trying to explain to him, "No, no, no, no, get out of there, get
> out of there, you've got to have this on and this on." He didn't
> understand a word I was saying, and I was trying to explain to
> him how to clean the room properly and safely. And I gave up.

Lack of opportunities to speak with colleagues because of a lack of time and the need to maintain physical distance increased workers' sense of miscommunication and lack of information. A housekeeper said she had repeatedly asked for debriefings or huddles, even virtually, so her team could be informed and support each other, but no action had been taken. In response, she brought in radios on her own initiative so her colleagues could at least talk to each other while maintaining physical distance.

CONCLUSION

An interviewee reflected on the first year of COVID-19 in LTC:

> I think the challenge that people had is the vulnerabilities
> of the sector were always there, it's just the pandemic magnified
> the cracks that were already in the system. And to try and fix
> something in such a short period of time and in a state of
> emergency is extraordinarily difficult. I don't think it's for
> want of trying, I think everyone is sincere in their efforts. But
> I also think it will take a sustained focus after the pandemic
> is over to fix what's broken.

The pre-COVID-19 vulnerabilities in the LTC sector meant that the women who staffed it were on the front lines of the pandemic, sometimes without the basic "weapons," like PPE and information, to keep themselves safe. Like soldiers, they witnessed unprecedented deaths and experienced daily threats of violence. Many were already on the verge of burnout and emotional exhaustion because of unsustainable workloads. Then they were exposed to the moral distress of watching the residents suffer alone, restricted in their ability to provide care by protocols and staffing shortages. Their grief directly affected their health and ability to provide care to their own families, but they had little time or meaningful opportunities to address it. While many managers tried to find ways to support staff and relay experiences to decision-makers, the typical style of emergency response – command-and-control – combined with pre-existing weakness in the sector, inhibited such efforts. However, while many LTC workers felt neglected and ignored, they also found innovative ways to connect with each other, and with residents and families.

COVID-19 has shone a light on the LTC crisis in Canada, with those working in it being both celebrated as heroes and vilified for the poor conditions in some facilities. The voices here suggest a deep level of caring by the women working in the sector, a degree of caring that negatively affected their own well-being. Considering the care these women demonstrated, it is worth listening to their advice on how to reform the sector. In particular, they suggested increasing the length of sick leave and standardizing sick leave policies for everyone working in the sector; concerted efforts to address violence and racism, including educating residents, workers, and employers; mandated job security guidelines that standardize wages, benefits, and allocation of work hours across care facilities; subsidized, accessible childcare services for LTC workers that meet the demands of shift work; comprehensive coverage for counselling, physical therapy, and recreation services for those working in LTC; and media strategies that promote public awareness of LTC workers as essential providers and highlight their ongoing challenges and inequities.

3

Masters of Disguise

Teachers

We've become masters of disguise. We present to our community
and our students as though we've done this a million times.

Middle school teacher

INTRODUCTION

On 15 March 2020, in response to the growing COVID-19 pandemic,
the Province of Alberta announced the closure of all schools and daycares, a lockdown that would last the rest of the school year. Over the
summer, as scientific understanding of COVID-19 increased and case
numbers declined, the decision was made to reopen schools, with the
option of online learning available to those families who chose it. Most
students and teachers returned to the classroom in September 2020
for a school year like no other. COVID-19 case numbers quickly began
to rise again, leading to secondary school closures in November 2020
and all schools shifting to online learning for the first few weeks
of 2021. While such measures led to a temporary reduction in cases,
numbers began to rise again in the spring with at first isolated and
then province-wide school closures in May 2021.

While numerous studies have analyzed the effects of COVID-19 on
students' education, few have considered the experiences of and effects
on teachers. A survey of Canadian teachers in April and June 2020
showed increasing burnout and cynicism (Sokal et al. 2020). A study
in BC found that teachers were anxious about student safety and

worried about supporting both online and face-to-face learning (MacDonald and Hill 2022). The same study found that teachers struggled with balancing teaching and personal commitments at home. In this chapter, I argue that teachers served as the, often unrecognized, home front – protecting students (and their own families) not only from a virus that spreads most easily in crowded rooms, but also from the secondary effects of the pandemic, such as increased anxiety and lost learning opportunities.

Few studies on COVID-19 and teaching in Canada, and few of those on teachers and previous health crises such as SARS and HINI, explicitly consider the gendered nature of teaching and how teachers' gender roles might affect their experiences of working during a public health crisis. Yet the field is distinctly feminized, with over 84 per cent of all primary teachers in Canada identifying as women (Statistics Canada 2018). Elsewhere, such as in Italy, research has shown that female teachers experienced a higher risk of negative mental health effects than male teachers (Matiz et al. 2020). A study from Chile found that female teachers experienced more negative effects on their quality of life, including work exhaustion and lower engagement with students, than male teachers (Lizana et al. 2021). This chapter explores the experiences of women teachers in Alberta, Canada, asking how their gender roles at work and home shaped their experiences of the pandemic.

In fall 2020, recognizing the lack of research on the experiences of women teachers and school leaders (which includes principals and vice-principals) in Alberta, the Alberta Teachers' Association (ATA) reached out to me and asked if I would be interested in conducting focus groups and interviews with women educators. Naturally, I agreed, and we held three focus groups during the ATA Women in Leadership Summit in March 2021, with two more the following week. In an effort to learn from a variety of experiences and incorporate intersectional analysis, focus groups were organized as follows:

- teachers from rural schools (six participants);
- teachers from Edmonton area schools (seven participants);
- teachers from Calgary area schools (six participants);
- school leaders (six participants); and
- teachers who identified as Indigenous or as racialized (four participants).

To better understand the policy context and key themes that emerged from the focus groups, I also conducted ten individual semi-structured interviews with school leaders and superintendents in May 2021. I asked participants to reflect on the 2020 to 2021 school year, but at times the discussion returned to the initial lockdown in spring 2020. All participants identified as women except one interviewee, who identified as a man. I shared the preliminary results with the ATA, refining the analysis through discussions and presentations.

This research occurred within a tense educational climate in Alberta. Alberta's education system remains one of the lowest funded in the country, with real per-pupil funding having declined by 15 per cent since 2013 (ATA 2022). Jason Kenney, the premier at the time of this research, was described as "spoiling for a fight with provincial teachers," with one of his first directives being to develop a new curriculum to avoid "failed pedagogical fads or political agendas in the classroom" (quoted in Fawcett 2021). The new curriculum has since been described as not only representing "the moral success story of liberal democracy coupled with market capitalism" but also forcing outdated pedagogic approaches on teachers (Bennett 2021). While the roll-out of this curriculum was postponed due to COVID-19, the threat of the added work of implementing it and widespread concern about how it would affect students' education hung over teachers and school educators. Similarly, many of the challenges respondents spoke of, such as a chronic substitute-teacher shortage and lack of access to child care, reflect a larger context of limited investment in social support and care infrastructure in the province, which has suffered from a downturn in the fossil fuel industries it previously relied on. While the interviews and focus groups did not explore political views or reflections on the political climate, this broader context shaped teachers' and school leaders' career and care conditions during the pandemic.

THE QUADRUPLE BURDEN

A school principal described an interaction with her therapist before the return to school in September 2020: "The first question she asked me in my therapy session was, 'What's the worst thing that could happen? My answer was, 'Someone could die on my watch.'" In addition to adapting to online and hybrid learning, teachers and school leaders became responsible for designing and implementing public health protocols. In their research with teachers following the initial COVID-19 lockdown, MacDonald and Hill (2022) found that returning to school in the fall of 2020 created high levels of anxiety for educators, who were concerned about how to keep children apart, felt safety guidelines were unclear, and worried about the potential for further closures and transitions to online learning. Research participants expressed similar concerns about the start of the school year. As one teacher noted, "[B]eing responsible for health and safety of other people's children in the middle of a global pandemic is heavy and anxiety-inducing." Principals and teachers felt this responsibility came with little guidance from Alberta Health Services and the Ministry of Education. A principal noted, "I think that a lot of teachers felt some concern with the PPE when we first started. Also, there was a lot of confusion about the return to school entry plans. We were basically required to create them on our own, kind of last minute." Additional cleaning and monitoring for sickness added to teacher workloads. A school leader described teachers in her school as "working their butt off sanitizing these desks a million times, they're watching for every little sniffle underneath the masks, and they're just exhausted by the extra work other than teaching and I think that's the biggest impact we've had." The need to protect against and respond to an unfolding pandemic continued throughout the school year as new information emerged, guidelines changed, and waves of infections followed. As one teacher reflected, having to "be adaptive and flexible, and to problem solve and to be nimble, and to learn new skills while trying to provide instruction for everybody else who is learning new skills has been extraordinarily difficult." While teachers were quick to note that "teachers aren't afraid of hard work," the context of constant change and uncertainty led to feelings of never being prepared or fully able to protect themselves or their students.

School leaders, in particular, were responsible for implementing COVID-19 protocols within their schools and communicating them to families. Many leaders expressed feelings of responsibility for COVID-19 outbreaks and felt that cases in their schools reflected on their performance. One principal described a "perceived community pressure that you'll do everything you can to keep them safe, means that if somebody ends up not safe, it must be your fault. And that's a heavy load to carry." Principals felt they were literally asking people to trust them with their and their children's lives: "[N]ow I'm introducing myself to staff in August and saying, hi … please trust me with your life; come on into the building with 160 other people." They noted that while being in decision-making roles enabled them to develop policies tailored to their specific school's needs, it was also "a great way of passing off responsibility." Developing and communicating public health protocols added to stress and management burdens. Another school leader noted that during the first few months of the school year, "every decision we were called out on." This work was also time-consuming. One principal revealed that she had to call parents every time COVID-19-related information changed: "The other challenge we have is that we have so many families who do not speak English at home. And so, you send documents, and they may be translated, but some of our families don't read in their home language either. It's much easier for us to phone, because there's usually a higher level of conversational English that we can get by on."

In the event of a COVID-19 exposure, school leaders were responsible for calling potential contacts and relaying information on isolation and testing. One school leader shared "a typical day" during the pandemic:

> For example, today I had five bus kids, well that just threw my whole morning so I couldn't deal with anything on my desk this morning because I had five bus kids who are close contacts sitting in classrooms and they just got identified. I'm isolating kids, I'm putting them in spots, calling parents, settling those kids' nerves because when they hear they're close contacts they automatically think they're getting something shoved up their nose and they're crying, and they're scared, right. That was the whole morning this morning, so all the things I had planned this morning are going to get done this evening or tomorrow.

Another principal explained:

> I got the call personally yesterday at 11, I had to be at the school at noon, didn't leave till 3 p.m., so that was my Sunday. This is typical of every school administrator right now, having to go to their school, that principal was just on the phone right now they got a call last night at 10:15 p.m., had to be at the school by 10:30, done calls at one o'clock in the morning.

The possibility of getting a call at any time affected school leaders' ability to disconnect when not working. They described the anxiety of "waiting every minute on a weekend for the phone call to say you have a case of COVID in your school." Another noted that she "can't separate home and work anymore. And maybe that's too much. I have to be on call all the time." Similarly, a school leader explained, "You know, at night I'll go to bed, and I'll be thinking, OK, if this staff member is positive then I'm contact tracing in my head before I even go to sleep at night." While school leaders were willing, recognizing their leadership responsibility in an extraordinary circumstance, such work took a toll on their well-being: "As an administrator, you know that your time is going to be, like, you don't have an eight to three job, or an eight to five job; you have to work evenings, you're on weekends. But most of that, in a typical year, you would know ahead of time. Now you're constantly on call." Another described the constant stress of the year as: "I feel like I'm on this raft in the middle of the ocean and there's sharks constantly swimming around me, just getting closer. Sometimes they're getting closer and closer and then boom, we've got a case. That's kind of what it feels like sometimes."

Levels of stress were amplified by the emotional labour of communicating bad news to others. A principal described the compassion that was required to make contact tracing calls:

> You're having conversations with staff that they need to quarantine, and a hundred parents that they need to quarantine again and go get a COVID test done. They're conversations where you need to be emotionally invested too, and you need to be caring for them and be sensitive and compassionate.

Even when not contact tracing, school leaders had to field calls from parents:

> So not only have we had to do these contact tracing calls, you're getting calls all the time when numbers start to go up, where parents just need reassurance. And they're asking for you to tell them what to do and we can't tell them what to do so that's taxing too because those conversations are taking ten, twelve, thirteen minutes a call.

Conversations about exposures and quarantines were often emotional as parents became fearful and anxious about their own workloads. School leaders had to deal with these emotions compassionately and effectively while noting they didn't have answers to many of the questions parents were asking (such as "How am I going to work with my kid at home?").

Though they didn't have the same contact tracing responsibilities as school leaders, teachers also reported high emotional labour demands. A middle school teacher described a recent afternoon,

> I was trying to sort of finish up the day. A student popped in who had been unable to come in for a week and he needed to share some, you know, really powerful struggles, and you know, I wanted to be there for him. And so that started taking my day longer. And then I was walking out with my colleague, and she was telling me about her life and where things were at for her, and I was being an emotion[al] support there. And we were literally walking into the parkade and this teacher starts pulling out of her parking spot, sees us, pauses, opens the window with tears in her eyes needing to communicate her struggle that day. And I'm looking at my watch thinking, OK it's 5:30, you know, my family needs me too. And everybody's just on such a low-key level of stress, with the spikes of big stresses, and needing each other for community and communion to be able to work through some of the stuff. And so yes, it would be lovely if we could set those boundaries, but they don't exist because crisis and chaos, you know, doesn't always adhere to any sort of schedule.

Previous research has documented the prevalence of emotional labour within female-dominated professions, such as teaching, and that this work is rarely recognized and often undervalued (Isenbarger and Zembylas 2006). Teachers are often expected to provide emotional and physical care at schools without being recognized or compensated for this work (Ismael et al. 2021). Their emotional investment in their students' well-being is often manipulated to push them to work to the point of fatigue and burnout (Chatelier and Rudolph 2018). Teachers described how the COVID-19 context increased emotional labour demands requiring "emotional heavy lifting" and "smoothing over other peoples' anxiety." The emotional needs of students were often acute. One teacher recounted how a student had interrupted an online class to express suicidal thoughts. Others expressed concerns about increased rates of violence within homes, economic hardship, and substance use related to COVID-19, which "put a huge, huge pressure and stress on the schools, on the teachers and administrators."

Teachers frequently mentioned the effort that went into trying to maintain a sense of calm or normalcy for students within the pandemic context. One teacher explained, "[W]e're trying to create as much normalcy as we can for our students and families," and another described "the expectation that we're bringing the calm and not amplifying the chaos." This took a substantial effort. One teacher joked, "I was just thinking, we've become masters of disguise. We present to our community and our students as though we've done this a million times." This caring and emotional labour was recognized as beneficial and essential by school leaders and superintendents, one of whom explained, "One thing that I have seen that's been really positive this year is the increased desire in staff to build relationships with students. And so, because they are so concerned about them, they're really working hard to keep them engaged with school, regardless of whether it's from the point of view of just the teacher or I guess more in a caring, concerned kind of way."

Teachers and school leaders described how the increased workloads and emotional labour at school necessarily affected their home life, commenting, "[O]f course you take it home with you." One principal noted, "I go home every day very exhausted because I'm constantly trying to reassure staff or students or families." They also noted that they faced increasing demands on their time and energy at home: "[M]y primary concern will still be the school, but I am also primarily responsible for the logistics of my family and then I'm trying to do both of those." Increased care demands within their homes and families fell primarily on women due to gendered roles and norms. One educator noted a difference in how her children treated her and her husband: "[W]hen my husband, who is a teacher, shuts the door, they won't bug him. But they'll come – someone might come through that door at any moment and come ask me for something, right ... because as the mom you're the go-to person." A superintendent identified a similar trend of female teachers trying to balance child care and professional responsibilities:

And one of the things that I'm seeing in my system is that they are also the caregiver in their home. When their children are at home or there is a requirement, it is often the woman, the educator, that is taking leave and going home. Where their partner is perhaps remaining in their job. It is the teacher that's going home and trying to teach online and care for the kids in the home. I think that there is a disproportionate responsibility to manage the global pandemic placed on women educators.

These conflicting responsibilities were particularly pronounced when educators' own children had to isolate or experienced school/childcare closures, which was not an unusual or one-off experience. One school leader noted that she "had some staff members that had to quarantine up to three times for upwards of ten to fourteen days. So again, if you're living with a family, [you're] basically stuck in [your] bedroom trying to manage your teaching assignments, stay away from your family, isolating, manage the day-to-day domestic responsibilities of being a parent or having food on the table or whatever else it is that you're responsible for." Many mothers said that, because they were teachers, they were also often the parent designated to support their children in online schooling: "When I had my little people at home, I would work until five, go home, make dinner and then I would teach from seven until ten. I would be prepping every day at school to go home and teach them every night. Which was exhausting." Another noted, "I was the one that was doing like everything with her schooling, making sure, OK, I've got this printed for her, you know ... My husband, I would say my husband was useless at the time just because it was like it's just, you know, up to the mother to make sure the schooling's done and doing all that part of it."

COVID-19 prevented many women from reaching out to their networks for help in coping with added childcare responsibilities. One teacher explained that her fear of transmitting COVID-19 impeded accessing family support: "Our family childcare model had been based on grandparents. That was a real luxury to have in non-COVID times, but it wasn't sustainable in COVID times." Another noted, "I can't even put into words how not having a babysitter for a four-year-old in over a year has changed the landscape of life at home." In addition, the awareness that everyone else was also struggling meant that previous community support systems were scarce:

Women are good at helping other women, right. In a good year I'm dropping off cooking on your doorstep, and I've got someone who drops off cookies on my doorstep, or I will take your kids on Saturday afternoon, so you can go to the gym on your own. The problem is, we're all in the same boat. So, the ways in which women have helped each other since the beginning of time, isn't doable right now, because everyone is struggling – I can't ask, because I know you're drowning too, and I can't help you, because I'm drowning too.

As this teacher noted, women have dealt with previous crises by sharing care burdens. COVID-19 negated this coping strategy on many levels (Krase et al. 2021).

The inability to rely on family and social networks particularly affected unpartnered mothers. One said, "I have taken a lot of the brunt on things and it's different, it is different from like having a two-parent or a two-caregiver family. Because at least you can trade off, you can say, you know what, I'm reading a book, I'm having a, I'm going to go for a walk, I'm doing this or that … There is no break, there's no break, there's been no break since the pandemic started." An unpartnered vice-principal described her usual morning:

So, as I drive to work when my kids are getting themselves to school, I'm like talking through getting them out the door for ten minutes, which for all the moms out there, you just let them do it. You don't talk to them while they're doing it because then you have panic attacks on the way to work. So, I stopped calling. But to live with that and have no one else here to get them out the door, and then be you know also getting anxious about the people forming at my door as I walk in with all of their emergencies, is a lot. Right. And then to walk in and look like I have answers and solutions while my child you know can't find her gloves or her – you know her brother isn't helping her or something.

Unpartnered educators who are mothers faced impossible choices about which responsibilities – home or work – to prioritize.

In addition to childcare responsibilities, many educators also had elder-care responsibilities. One teacher explained:

Since my father passed away several years ago, I have tried to make Saturday a committed day to go see my mother. And because of this year, and how things are, and concerns over her health and well-being, it's not only a matter now of when do I see my mother, but it's also a matter of if she needs groceries.

It's also a matter now of if she needs whatever, I'm the person that is doing that for her reliably ... So, there are greater home demands, there are greater professional demands.

Educators' professional risk of infection caused conflicts about whether they should continue to provide care and then increase their elder's risk of infection or withhold care and further isolate the elder. Previous research by the ATA (2020) found that 71 per cent of teachers and school leaders were moderately to extremely concerned about bringing the virus home from school, and the participants in this study shared those concerns. An Indigenous teacher explained that she was the primary care provider to her parents and was therefore anxious about ensuring their health: "[M]y parents are elderly, my dad is seventy years old and my mom is sixty-six, and I know Indigenous people we're a little bit more susceptible." She was constantly negotiating how to ensure her parents had necessities and emotional support while reducing physical contact. Another teacher noted, "I do live with my mother ... She is over sixty-five. And so, you know, one of my stresses is that being in the school environment, that I could bring COVID home to her." Teachers and school leaders recognized that COVID-19 did not respect boundaries between home and work and could easily be transmitted across care responsibilities.

BEING ESSENTIAL

Despite taking on public health roles and living with the risk of infection and its secondary effects on unpaid care responsibilities, teachers were not prioritized for COVID-19 vaccines. At the time of the focus groups and interviews (spring 2021), Alberta had begun vaccinating the general public. While healthcare workers were prioritized, teachers, despite being designated as essential workers and fulfilling essential public health and caregiving roles, were not. Instead, they were being vaccinated according to age on the same schedule as the general public. To many, this lack of prioritization symbolized a lack of recognition of their essential service. A teacher expressed:

Our government decided not to consider us essential enough for a vaccination, so it was like then adding salt to the wound. So, we're keeping your economy going because we're babysitting your kids and we're keeping them in school, but you don't think we are special enough to maybe be bumped up the line a little bit to get the vaccination so that we can still come to school.

Others described not being prioritized for vaccination as "a slap in the face," noting that early access was not just about protecting teachers' health but also demonstrating that they were valued essential workers and recognizing the risks they were taking.

> To say there's no vaccine – to not say a thing about vaccines for teachers, as an example, is one thing. To say, we see you, we understand the risks that you're taking each day, we understand the perceived effect that that has on your life, and the impact on your families, and we will get you vaccines when we can. I think even if it doesn't change the date that they become available for teachers, it changes the whole – oh, well, okay, thanks, you do see me.

Lack of vaccine prioritization was seen as the ultimate example of disregard for teachers' contributions and the risk they assumed.

Many teachers also commented on an overall lack of support and flexibility for managing the multiple demands placed upon them. An Indigenous teacher and single mother noted, "There is nothing that I can see, like extra support ... I haven't, like no one has contacted specifically, like no one has reached out to me based on, you know, being a single mother during this time, no one's reached out to me being like an Indigenous educator at this time, there's been nothing." While teachers did have access to leave if they needed to isolate or care for family members in isolation, there was ambiguity about what to do when their paid leave was exhausted. One respondent revealed that they had three family sick days, which was insufficient in the context of COVID-19, and she felt it perpetuated the "whole notion around your job is far more important than your family." Similarly, teachers' experiences about what type of flexibility was allowed varied. One teacher noted that her administrators allowed her to leave early on the days she had to pick her child up from daycare. Another respondent recounted that when her child's daycare closed due to an exposure, she was told to "figure it out or quit."

Many educators felt unable to take leave when their care responsibilities became overwhelming due to a province-wide substitute-teacher shortage, which meant their colleagues would be overburdened with their work if they took time off. A lack of trained teachers (reflecting ongoing under-investment in the sector) meant that many school districts, particularly in rural areas, did not even have enough substitute teachers to manage pre-pandemic teacher absences. The pandemic not only increased the frequency of teacher absences, because those with symptoms and exposures had to isolate, but also reduced supply, because many substitute teachers decided to only serve one or two schools to reduce their risk of exposure. When substitute teachers were not available, which was often the case, gaps had to be filled within the school. One school leader noted,

> The impact for staff is that whenever you don't have coverage for your building, you are then using internal coverage – who has a prep period, who has a piece of time, who has a lunch break, who has a recess break, who has time, which is intended over the course of that day to allow them to recharge, to make sure that they have the energy that they need ... I haven't met a teacher that hasn't rallied to help their colleagues and to provide internal coverage. Teachers have huge hearts, and they are so giving. The issue becomes, certainly for a system like ours where we've had week after week after week after week after week, of not having appropriate numbers of substitutes.

Like other essential professions, staff shortages prevented teachers from fulfilling their other essential role as a care provider at home.

In high schools, teachers often responded to the substitute shortage by shifting to online teaching; if a teacher had to quarantine, they would instruct virtually from their home. As one school leader described, "[A]t one point we had fourteen teachers away, and so to bring fourteen subs in, we couldn't find fourteen subs, and so then we ended up changing the system. Then the poor kids, if their teacher was quarantined, it's like, you guys, you're not quarantined, but your class is going to be online for the next two weeks, because we couldn't find subs." Virtual learning, described as "a gong show" and "no end of confusion," was recognized as a poor solution for both the students, who lost out on in-person interactions, and the teachers, who had to work from home while dealing with the personal challenges of isolating and potential COVID-19 illness. One teacher described online learning as follows:

It's twenty or thirty children on the other end of the computer that need computer assistance that can't find their login, that are having volume problems that need help. All of those problems need to be resolved. While a teacher has things going on at home that involve the rest of their world. And in addition, then trying to teach a lesson that they probably spent weeks getting organized, ready to teach in the classroom. And with no notice, now need to turn that into somehow doing it in an engaging way online.

In such cases, teachers were expected to fulfill both their essential roles – professional and personal – simultaneously.

While teachers did not feel recognized and supported by educational leadership outside of their divisions, they did comment on the importance of receiving tokens of appreciation from colleagues, students, and parents. One primary school teacher mentioned that a high school teacher had sent her school pizza at lunch to recognize that they were still working in the classroom while the secondary school had shifted online. Another noted that a student leadership class had taken on the task of sending thank-you notes to teachers. Others commented on food and gifts from parents and local businesses. One school leader described how such tokens helped teachers "feel seen," reinforcing that their contribution to the response was recognized: "It doesn't have to be big, or a trophy, but it's those emotional pieces, and I think it moves us even more when it comes systemically, or it comes from a supervisor, a colleague." They further noted that the interruptions to schooling had created greater appreciation for teachers and the school system in general, "And I think that staff and students have both developed a greater appreciation for school. So, the students are happy to be in school."

MENTAL WELLNESS, MORAL DISTRESS, AND BURNOUT

An ATA survey conducted in September 2020 found that 87 per cent of teachers and school leaders reported being exhausted at the end of each day. Teachers explained, "I as a teacher, I mean I graduated in '02, I have never been as tired as I have been this year. I call it teacher pandemic tired. I'm exhausted. By the end of the day, I don't even want to do anything. Between the pandemic stress, being micromanaged, it's exhausting." Many teachers noted that despite being exhausted, they had difficulty sleeping.

> I don't think I've slept really well since last March 16th. Because every single day I drive in to work and I wonder is this the day we're going to get another Alberta Health Services call? Is this a day that we're going to get the call and that's going to be another six hours of our team having to deal with that ... it's sort of that humming constant stress of what is about to happen that is – and that's why I said overwhelming and exhausting.

Administrators reflected that "the cracks are starting to be noticed on educators and then what will be the physical result out of that down the road, because they're not taking care of themselves, they're just taking care of everyone else." Numerous women similarly worried about the long-term physical effects of the high stress and anxiety they were experiencing daily.

Many teachers expressed moral distress at their inability to ensure that students met educational goals and at their struggles to manage care responsibilities at home. Much like healthcare providers when they have to care for patients without adequate supplies, teachers expressed a sense of helplessness. A teacher who worked with children with special needs noted:

> One of the hardest things that I had to face was, I worried about my kids. I worried, like, many of my kids are autoimmune compromised and so I worried, like, would they be okay. And then it was one of those, like, they don't socialize as it is, you know, before COVID. And now, having them being stuck in their homes, how are they going to be okay, you know, were they going to be okay? How could I make that, you know, their life be normal, and trying to achieve that? How was I supposed to support their families when I couldn't see them?

Teachers felt compelled to continue to provide high-quality education and support to students, even when they were unable to due to COVID-19 restrictions. A school principal reflected, "I think that teachers always feel – or often, I would say – they feel ... the moral obligation to ensure that their students are educated and educated well. And during COVID, because of the way that things had been handled, I think that there's a feeling of not being able to do their best work, or perhaps failure in some way." Many educators spoke about the challenge of ensuring student preparedness to meet provincial standards and felt responsible if such standards were not met. Being unable to meet student needs led to a sense of failure: "I would say it's the constant unknown and trying to plan for that, and always feeling like you're failing."

Moral distress extended into educators' personal lives, especially when their occupational commitment infringed on their ability to meet their care responsibilities at home. A large-scale study on teacher experiences during the COVID-19 pandemic showed that educators with children in their household experienced greater increases in anxiety than those without (Allen et al. 2020). Stress was caused by a mismatch between job demands and job resources, ever-changing circumstances, and a sense of moral responsibility (Sokal et al. 2020). Teachers noted that it was simply impossible to meet both career and care goals: "[P]hysically there are not enough hours in the day to do everything that you ask of working mums, like, things in the home." As a result, many respondents felt they were failing as parents to (somewhat) manage their professional workload: "I feel like I'm spending more time with the school kids than my own kids. I'm at school and worrying about them more than I am my own children at home." This led to feelings of guilt, such as, "It will take me quite some time to get over the wrongness and the guilt of not parenting my own kids in the height of the pandemic from March till June." Mothers expressed anxiety about the quality of their children's care and education: "We have one child who is kind of old enough to leave on her own. But there's stresses around that. Like we don't feel like we're endangering her, but you know she needs more guidance, she needs more attention and she's not able to be social with friends right now. I think the weight of that has been heavy." Not being able to strike a balance between the needs of children at home and students at school has caused educators to feel they were constantly failing on one front or another. As discussed by one principal, "I think it's always feeling, again, like, they're letting someone down, and right now it's either they're letting their students down, or their biological children – the human that they birthed." This in turn led to feelings of helplessness: "I felt really defeated. I felt like I wasn't doing a good enough job, I felt like a loser. I was at a loss, how was I supposed to help my kids, and I felt like I was losing every day."

The prevalence of distress – because of the impossibility of meeting both students' and their children's needs – was linked to increased burnout. One teacher predicted, "I actually foresee larger administrator burnout. I'm so happy I have a fantastic administrator, but I see what she has to do in a day, and it's just not humanly possible. Like this has encapsulated her life in every way." Superintendents worried about attrition within their division: "We're at a terrible risk for burnout of educators. We have people requesting leaves for next year, we have an increase in medical leaves that are occurring. We have individuals that we anticipated taking a leave next year asking for early leave. As a superintendent, that is probably one of my greatest worries is the health and well-being of our system. And will we have adequate staff going forward?" Many educators noted that they had lost their passion for teaching:

> I feel discouraged … we don't talk as much about student
> learning anymore. Which is, we're supposed to be instructional
> leaders. We talk about safety protocol[s] and implementing rules,
> which obviously are really important. That would be one
> piece – it's removed the reason why I do the work that I do.

The overwhelming focus on COVID-19 protocols and the prioritization of health over education reduced teachers' sense of the kind of return they were getting on the time and energy they invested in their work.

Within this context, teachers and school leaders felt there was limited mental health support. One school leader noted that despite all the focus on maintaining physical health through COVID-19 protocols, little attention was paid to maintaining mental health:

> I think that the piece that they left out was the people piece. There
> were lots of rules about safety … but there was very little, read
> zero, indication of how do we support mental health and wellness.
> It gets discussed at every meeting and they say things like, call
> [mental health service], and so on. But nothing in terms of how
> do we support our teachers, our support staff, our students, our
> families who are going through many crises during this time.

Some educators had sought counselling through the mental health services provided to all ATA members. Others sought support from in-school counsellors, who were seen as helpful but overworked.

A number of teachers commented that professional development days dedicated to self-care were highly beneficial. Professional development days are typically days students don't come to school so that teachers can engage in training. During the 2020–21 school year, some schools decided that instead of attending workshops or training events, teachers could use the day for self-care. One teacher explained:

> We had a Pro-D day for the district; it was a Friday in November and we were all talking about it and it was going to be virtual, etc. And then all of a sudden we got an email, full-staff email from our superintendent saying, "You guys have worked hard, you're stressed; we're just teachers. It's going to be a – it's a non-day, stay home. We gave you a holiday." So, they took a Pro-D day and let us stay home, which – to get that one day off was remarkable, and we had a lot of teachers that – you know, it doesn't make up for everything but it showed that at least they understood that we're really, really trying.

The act of giving teachers a day to get caught up and take care of themselves was seen as both symbolically and practically significant, with many teachers commenting on how it provided a chance to "catch my breath."

In spring 2021, a teacher accurately predicted, "COVID-19 [is] not going to go away if everyone's being immunized. Those people whose family fell apart … they are still dealing with the after-effects of that for years and years to come. This is not just, oh well, okay, we're all immunized and we're just going to go on tomorrow. There's going to be a lot of residual effects, for sure." While the teacher quoted here was focusing on the well-being of students, her distress also described the residual effects on teachers' well-being and mental health. Much like soldiers who continue to suffer post-traumatic stress disorder (PTSD) decades after a conflict has ended, teachers may continue to process the trauma they experienced and witnessed during the pandemic long after it's over.

POWER

One of the most surprising outcomes of the focus groups with teachers and school leaders, particularly considering the findings above, was that half the respondents reported feeling inspired to take on new career or leadership responsibilities (see figure 2.1). Similarly, administrators noted that teachers and school leaders had stepped up in response to the pandemic: "You know, teachers could say, I have no time right now, I can't even talk about these big things about school. And in fact, I think I've seen an increase in engagement." When asked why, in a context of an increased workload at school and home and high levels of stress, they wanted to take on more responsibility, teachers noted that the skills and abilities they had to offer were needed: "I feel like I can maybe help in ways that we're needing moving forward, and I think that is actually where a lot of – we as women can step up, moving forward, in light of all the challenges that we face in this pandemic, for sure." Participants noted an urgent need for leadership that could provide emotional support and understand the caregiving challenges teachers were facing, the skills and knowledge they felt women leaders could offer. One teacher commented on how her role as someone who cares for others positively affected her leadership ambitions: "I am that person who feels that caregiver need for your colleagues, and when [it] looks like colleagues are getting beaten on sometimes, it's, well, how do I fix that? Well, you have to fix that from inside the system. Which system can I fix that through?" Others noted a new appreciation for skills often recognized as feminine, "[T]hose soft skills, the more care-giver type of mentality, I suppose, is very much being relied on right now, as people are recognizing the stress levels. And it is that kind of caregiving that's getting a lot of people through." A superintendent noted that women were indeed acting on identified needs:

What I'm seeing in our women leaders is a real strong effort to try and support the emotional and mental health of the staff and the students and the families. That has been a dominant theme in our conversations, about what are they doing? How are they doing? How are they outreaching? What are they dropping off or texting or messaging or phoning? There's this heightened support network as a result from the women leading in our system.

Several participants expressed an interest in updating their qualifications to become school counsellors, which requires a master's degree, recognizing the urgent need for mental health services.

Teachers also recognized that the pandemic had created more accessible online options for gaining additional qualifications. For example, one teacher shared that online programming enabled her to pursue a master's degree:

I think just the availability and opportunity is presented differently now because of COVID. For example, I've been wanting to pursue a master's for a while, and now, just because things are so available online, and I have a young family, and I have an office set up at home now, it's a little bit more accessible for me, just because of the way that the world is right now. And it might not have been something that I would have been able to as actively pursue even a year ago. Just something as simple as that has been helpful. It's a positive outcome from this situation.

Others made similar statements: "It has also inspired me then to start looking at like applying for a master's and kind of working my way up possibly to an administrative position. And so just being able to connect that way with other people, although challenging and exhausting, it has inspired me to kind of become a better leader." Not having to travel to major cities, like Calgary or Edmonton, and being able to learn from home reduced the barriers teachers faced to pursuing further education themselves.

Others benefited from more accessible professional development opportunities, describing themselves as "at the highest place in my teaching trajectory" due to online learning opportunities. One educator noted: "What I have truly enjoyed is all the online free professional development and things that you can just do, and then I don't have to go and have wine and listen to hockey with the same fellow down the hall all the time. I can have something else to do. I've learned all kinds of new things this year, and been able to explore some things in ways that I haven't been able to before." Shifting away from in-person networking and learning to online options created new opportunities for women with care responsibilities at home to pursue career development.

However, those leadership ambitions were also tempered by overwhelming workloads and a lack of support for unpaid care responsibilities. One principal felt that "there [are] a lot of women in leadership right now, this particular year saying there's no way. This is not my cup of tea." One participant similarly noted that COVID-19 "might make women take a step away from seeking leadership because this has been a lot for them. And it kind of reinforces them back into a recognition that they need to be the primary childcare provider even as a working woman and that stepping into leadership makes it more difficult for them." Teachers cited increased care work outside of school as especially

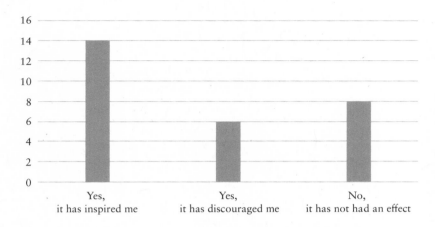

Figure 2.1 Focus group responses to poll question "Has the pandemic affected your career aspirations?"

discouraging them from pursuing or continuing in leadership. A woman who recently took on a new leadership position noted:

This is my second year as a vice-principal, and it really took the wind out of my sails. I was so excited when I got this job, and it was the year after I had a baby. I was, like I had a new baby, and I found a daycare, and I was going to be a school leader, and I was super excited. And went through, you know, 2019–20 in all of the not so greatness of it, but then I got here this year and I was ready to go, and then it's just like, it hits you.

Inability to work from home or judgment about working from home were further barriers to pursuing leadership opportunities. One superintendent noted, "We have a few principals who have young children, who are women, who they can't be in their school. If their children are isolated, they have to be at home. And they feel like the perception among the rest of their colleagues and even within their school community is that they're not doing their job." This perception was evidenced by another superintendent, who recounted,

I was speaking to you know a colleague of mine ... who is male, who I respect greatly, we were talking about somebody and sort of their career trajectory, and he said, "Well, I don't think they'd be considered for that position because they're mostly working from home right now." And I said, "Do you realize she has two little ones? Like that's her reality." And so, you know, I was glad to set him straight, but I don't think it occurred to him that that fell on her shoulders as a burden and that really that was the only way for their family to cope.

Witnessing the experiences of and judgment about women in leadership positions during COVID-19 also discouraged others from advancing their careers. A principal noted, "There are people who come to me and say, 'I never want to do this job, because this is not what I signed up for.'"

Women school leaders observed that it was often difficult to share these concerns with leadership in the educational sector. One principal noted, "[W]e'll get called to meetings. We're asked for input. But the decision is already made." Participants cited examples of requests denied to direct funding to mental health support or that school leaders be able to work from home as evidence of a lack of meaningful consultation. One school leader noted that despite most educators being mothers, space was not created for them to discuss their experiences as working parents or their concerns about school safety:

But there was no permission in the spring or summer for those of us with young kids at home, mums with young kids at home, in leadership roles, to speak up, to ask questions and to share our worries, so we've been quiet. We'd have a meeting and be very polite in the meeting and we would say, "Oh yes, we must be in schools, yes, they must be" ... But after the meeting, or quietly in the hallway, you know, somewhere else later you could say, "Are you terrified about coming back in August? Yeah, me too."

One participant commented on how this restricted effective decision-making, saying, "You know there is value in having the voice of leadership in such a female-dominated profession of a working mom. And oftentimes that's missing." Another noted,

I think policy, decisions, comments made, all those things you know they're through a lens of someone who is not living it. It's well intentioned. And often they have their own children and they're not clueless and out of touch and all of those things.

But a lot of them have never been a mom, and they're not the one with a four-year-old running around their ankles when they're trying to work. They don't have that lived experience. And they don't necessarily reach out to people who have had it. I think that would be a good.

In other words, listening to women's voices and experiences could have strengthened the response to COVID-19 in Alberta schools, and capitalized on, instead of frustrated, the ambitions of women educators to provide the highest standard of education and care possible.

CONCLUSION

During a school year like no other, teachers and school leaders, the vast majority of whom are women, not only strove to defend the home front, through public health measures and contact tracing, but also provided quality education in a context of constant uncertainty, alongside teaching their own children at home and caring for older relatives. They felt a deep sense of responsibility for the safety and well-being of their students and their families, an obligation further exemplified by the emotional labour they invested in prioritizing others' needs over their own. Their work burdens and care responsibilities were impossible to reconcile, leading to high levels of stress, feelings of failure, and guilt, with long-term implications for mental health and well-being.

Rather than being defeated by such burdens, many educators rose to the challenge, taking on the task of keeping schools safe and families functioning. Some recognized opportunities to advance their learning and leadership opportunities and seized them. However, this potential was threatened by a lack of support for women educators, particularly in managing both work and care responsibilities. Despite widespread evidence that workloads and care burdens were unmanageable and unsustainable, little effort was made to ease these burdens, but when tokens of recognition, flexible policies, and compassion for care responsibilities were offered, women educators truly appreciated them.

Without improved support for teachers, school leaders, students, and families, the risk of burnout continues to be real. Teachers and school leaders offered the following recommendations to ease the ongoing burden of COVID-19: flexibility to allow working from home where and when possible; a holistic approach to supporting teacher well-being, including paid care leave days; access to counselling and other supports; professional development days dedicated to COVID-19 recovery activities, such as how to support students who have experienced schooling gaps, mental wellness, and building community; resources to support women educators in pursuing career development, including support for care responsibilities that might restrict opportunities; ensuring diverse voices in decision-making; and developing equity policies to guard against discrimination based on gender, care responsibilities, or leave taken due to COVID-19. Educators noted that in the case of future pandemics, contact tracing should be the responsibility of public health professionals, not school leaders; additional emergency paid care leave should be provided, communicated, and standardized across the province; and on-site child care should be provided for those who have to be in the school building during widespread lockdowns.

4

Swimming in Quicksand

Nurses

I think a lot of the times people forget that we're not just nurses right, we're parents, we're mothers, we're daughters, we're grandchildren. And when you're a nurse, you're a nurse everywhere. You're not just a nurse when you go to work, you're nursing everybody in your life, and so it wasn't even like your due diligence to protect the people you cared for or to protect yourself, it was the huge responsibility of protecting your loved ones back at home.

COVID-19 ward nurse

When we conjure up the image of a frontline essential worker, many of us think of a nurse. We see a woman in scrubs and a mask, heroic in the face of sickness, death, and the body fluids most of us recoil from. We view the nurse as someone who is indefatigable, who can deploy a range of tools at once to defeat multiple threats from all directions. But this image is also deceptive. Nurses are human: they run out of energy; they feel emotional distress; they are not indestructible.

Many of the nurses whose experiences are recounted here not only provided COVID-19-related care but were also responding to the secondary health effects of the pandemic, such as increased overdoses from lethal drugs. The 90 per cent of nurses in BC who identify as women are also likely to have dependents at home, whose care and education needs increased during COVID-19. Nurses have been rightly celebrated as the heroes of the COVID-19 response, positioned as they are at the centre of all of these complex crises in hospitals, homes, and communities.

As with many of the feminized professions in this book, nursing was facing staffing shortages and high rates of burnout even before the pandemic. Pre-COVID-19 research showed that not having enough time to complete all their essential tasks due to their high workloads resulted in nurses being anxious and depressed, and losing sleep (MacPhee, Dahinten, and Havaei 2017). The pandemic only exacerbated the risk of burnout. A survey conducted by the BC Nurses' Union (BCNU) in fall 2021 stated that many nurses "were at a breaking point long before the COVID-19 pandemic, and the added stresses they have endured throughout this extensive public health emergency have greatly impacted their mental and physical health" (BCNU 2021, 3). Less research has been done on nurses' home life and unpaid care work before and during the pandemic, or how such responsibilities interacted with their multiple professional roles.

Through four focus groups and three semi-structured interviews with eleven nurses during January and February 2021, this chapter explores nurses' experiences not just as healthcare providers, but also as unpaid care providers, asking how the pandemic has affected nurses' well-being and the sustainability of the profession in BC. Some interviewees worked directly with COVID-19 patients, whereas others spoke of their experiences providing care to those facing other health crises, such as the opioid epidemic, and the overall challenges within the health system.

THE QUADRUPLE BURDEN

Nurses saw their workloads increase rapidly during the first few months of the pandemic because they had to stay up to date on the most current research, implement new and often changing protocols, increase cleaning, and ensure COVID-19-related care. One nurse explained, "Management would say "'Oh just look up the new policy' and it's like you scroll through fifty thousand things and it's like literally like I don't have time for that, I haven't even peed yet. I have to don and doff every five seconds and I'm sweating. I can't even see, like it was ridiculous." In particular, hospitals lacked nurses who knew how to intubate patients and were experienced in critical care, increasing the burden on those who did have those skill sets. Many described not having time to take breaks and as a result being "chronically dehydrated, with bladder infections, and starving, for the last half of our shifts." One nurse described her inability to get everything done within a shift: "Being expected to do our work, chart online, look after patients, and go on breaks – it's impossible. I just can't do it all. I end up staying later to chart. Everything is taking longer because of the pandemic, even just getting dressed up."

Not all the increases in workload were directly related to COVID-19. Nurses working with individuals who used substances or were unhoused saw their caseloads increase due to the higher pressures on equity-deserving populations and restricted access to community services, leading to increased social isolation, illness, and overdose. A community-based nurse explained:

> The acuity of my clients changed rather rapidly. There was a toxic drug supply, the borders were closed, clients were using toxic substances and due to stress, they relapsed on those substances. So, my caseload went completely sideways within about two weeks ... [Previously] we would have five to ten clients a week sent to my team. The first three weeks of the pandemic we had seventy-five referrals and that's on top of the caseload of thirty-nine clients that I was already carrying.

Nurses were providing some of the only available care at the heart of the COVID-19 and toxic drug supply crises. Reduced preventive and primary care services meant that those who did access care were often in acute need, and caseloads in the community clinics that remained open increased dramatically.

Although COVID-19 protocols sought to reduce risk, the constant change in guidelines increased nurses' anxiety and complicated their workflows. One nurse explained:

> It seems like things are perpetually changing but depending on our experiences. Like for example, my COVID patient coded, coded while I was in the room and with the respiratory therapist. And we had to kind of troubleshoot, how are we going to get the crash cart in the room? Because we don't want to contaminate the crash cart. So, we had it half in the room, half out. It was totally awkward. And so, we had to troubleshoot, while we were trying to run a code on this woman.

Another nurse reiterated that experience:

> Especially in those code situations where things are critically
> changing, or things are happening so fast. And then you add
> in COVID and it's like you're not only figuring out the code
> or what's going on; you're also figuring out am I wearing
> the proper PPE, has this person had the test, have they been
> swabbed, has it been back, are they pending ... On the medical
> floor, sometimes patients are there for quite a few days, and so
> they could have been COVID-swabbed, their precautions are
> down, and you don't know so you're trying to flip through
> the chart and figure it out.

The constant uncertainty that came with the changing procedures
increased both physical and mental workloads.

A number of nurses noted how "heartbreaking" it was to see social
media posts of people spending time with their families during lockdown, baking and crafting. In contrast, nurses had reduced time with
their families and struggled to arrange additional child care. Schools
and daycares were either only open for limited hours or completely
closed, and the child care provided to essential workers during lockdown did not correspond to most nurses' work hours. One nurse
explained that child care was available at her son's school from 8 a.m.
until 4 p.m., but she worked from 7 a.m. to 7 p.m. Health regulations
stated that only one parent should do drop-off and pickup, impossible
to arrange when both parents worked shift work. Nurses were reluc-
tant to rely on other family members to fill the care deficit, recognizing
that their risk of occupational infection would extend to any close
contacts – a well-founded fear because, after care aides in LTC, nurses
were the second most likely profession to contract COVID-19
(CIHI 2021a). One nurse said that her dad used to help care for her
son when she had to work, but this was no longer possible because he
was immunocompromised. Two nurses explained that due to the lack
of options, they had both gone part-time to be able to share child care.

Many expressed guilt about not having time to support their children's online schooling. A nurse explained, "My kids were supposed
to be getting home-schooled, and I was at work every day and I felt
like I was kind of sacrificing them, my own kids." Another nurse
described trying to help her kid with math via text at work: "My kid
sat home fending for himself texting me constantly that he has anxiety

trying to do math and I'm responding with a cellphone in a Ziploc bag to not get contaminated." The grades of another nurse's son slipped because she wasn't there to help him with his homework. And because he was in high school, her son didn't qualify for the support provided to kids of frontline workers. Because he was in his last year of school, she worried that her lack of support would affect his grades, which would prevent him from attending university.

Nurses expressed further concern about the physical and mental well-being of their children and their anxiety about providing enough comfort and support. A mother of a four-year-old son explained that she had planned on her son starting preschool in 2020, but due to the challenge of managing with her schedule, she had decided to keep a nanny employed. She was now concerned that her son was overweight due to a lack of exercise and was missing out on opportunities to learn social skills. One nurse described working six days a week, in twelve-hour shifts, so she felt she had "lost track of [her] son." She described how her son had changed:

> His life had changed drastically – he was no longer going to school or being active. He stayed up all night, slept all day, didn't eat properly. I wasn't able to home-school him. At the time I thought, "you know what, he's alive, it's the best I can do" but then became increasingly aware his mental health was suffering, it took me six months to get him back on track.

Nurses also recognized that the risk inherent in their work caused their children stress and anxiety. One nurse described showering and washing her scrubs as soon as she came home, while her kids waited impatiently, not understanding why they couldn't hug their mom right away. A nurse who contracted COVID-19 at work described feeling guilty about the effect it had on her children: "I was in isolation. They didn't know how I was doing. So, they were super stressed, anxious around is mom going to be OK?"

Some participants requested more flexible work schedules to accommodate unpaid care demands, but these requests were denied. One nurse had requested permission to do some of her paperwork from home:

> I could have juggled a bit more with my husband and it would have been a little less of a crisis situation sometimes. And it was totally unnecessary, I could have got my work done at different

hours of the day and it would have been fine for all of my patients. It would not have impacted their care at all, but they were so obsessed with time theft that they couldn't be flexible.

Another nurse described her request to work from home being "shot down." Another explained that her kids would cry when she left each morning, often causing her to be a few minutes late, for which she would be disciplined. A mental health nurse described being told to work from home, but not being provided with child care: "We're expected to work at the same capacity as if there is not a pandemic, including maintaining the same level of confidentiality, which means not parenting." When the nurse noted that such arrangements were impossible, especially as she didn't have a private room to work from, an email went out telling workers that if they were unable to balance doing their job from home and caring for their children, they were expected to take unpaid leave. Nurses had an overwhelming sense that they were expected to prioritize their paid work over their unpaid care work.

BEING ESSENTIAL

Nurses were initially celebrated as the stereotypical essential worker. They described receiving free food and gifts at the hospital almost daily during the first few months of the pandemic. However, such tokens tapered off quickly. Nurses working in COVID-19 wards or short-staffed units described working without time for breaks to eat or rest. In addition to this, management restricted access to refrigerators, dishwashers, microwaves, and other cooking spaces to decrease the transmissibility of COVID-19. One nurse noted, "We're healthcare heroes, but no. We're not actually treated as heroes by our actual employer. Like not like you want to be treated like a hero. If like you're expected to work on your break and all these other things that we're expected to do – we don't even have access to coffee and tea, or a fridge." Another noted that because she didn't have time to make her own food, she would often rely on the leftover food from patients' trays. One nurse working a COVID-19 ward said all she wanted was a microwave so she could heat up her lunch, noting that the coffee machine she was using had been provided, not by the employer, but by a compassionate doctor who had noticed her going without. Many described how the combination of stress plus the lack of a healthy diet had caused them to either gain or lose an unhealthy amount of weight and develop digestive problems, such as nausea and diarrhea.

Many nurses reported being stigmatized, particularly those working with COVID-19 patients or with populations seen to be at risk, such as those who used substances or were unhoused. One nurse recounted the stigma from other healthcare workers:

> I was saying how we were helping out a COVID patient or whatever that morning. And one of the people in the office had overheard me and had gone to the manager and said "Well, if she was dealing with a COVID-positive patient, why is she even in this office?" ... So, I even experienced my own stigma from another healthcare worker. And that wasn't the only time.

Nurses described having other families cancel playdates with their children and feeling isolated from friends due to their fears of infection. One nurse recalled that her grandmother, for whom she was the primary care provider, would casually mention that she had to be extra careful: "How are you going to feel if you know you give me COVID and you kill me?" Such actions and comments conflicted with the public celebrations of essential workers as heroes; instead, one nurse described being treated "like a leper."

Conversely, those who did not accept scientific information about COVID-19 often targeted nurses with conspiracy theories. Family and friends opposed to public health protections would often purposefully seek out nurses, questioning the severity of COVID-19 and the effectiveness of vaccines. Not only were nurses frustrated by the propagation of misinformation, they also felt that it invalidated the work they were doing and the risks they had undertaken. One explained, "To hear of all the conspiracy theories and to hear about the people thinking it's just a way for the government to control us and these anti-maskers ... It was just very disheartening and difficult to digest all of that misinformation and everything that was happening and then what I was actually experiencing every day." As opposition to COVID-19 measures increased, nurses often became the targets of verbal attacks and hate messages. They were sometimes being harassed on their way to work or while providing essential services, such as staffing vaccine clinics – a stark contrast to the way they had been celebrated at the start of the pandemic.

MENTAL WELLNESS,
MORAL DISTRESS, AND BURNOUT

A survey conducted in July 2020 showed that among 3,676 working nurses, 47 per cent met the criteria for PTSD, 38 per cent for anxiety, and 41 per cent for major depression (Stelnicki, Carleton, and Reichert 2020). The mental health challenges were largely attributed to a rapid increase in workload due to staff shortages, limited access to appropriate PPE, and concerns about infecting family and friends with COVID-19. Similarly, research elsewhere has found that nurses experienced moral distress in response to having to care for patients, including those who were dying, without family members present, and due to fears of transmitting COVID-19 to family and patients (Lake et al. 2022). As noted in the preceding sections, the nurses whose experiences are shared here described similar worries, including family safety and securing child care, increased workloads, fear of being infected and spreading COVID-19, and social isolation/stigma from the community.

Nurses faced repeated experiences of moral distress related to COVID-19 protocols, inhibiting their ability to provide timely and quality care. For example, previously if a patient crashed (experienced a sudden negative change in their status), the nurse would respond immediately with potentially life-saving procedures. In the context of COVID-19, however, when a patient crashed, the nurses had to shut the door and make sure they had their PPE on before going in to resuscitate them, causing a delay. One nurse recounted,

> It's just, it's upsetting because there's a few moments, on my last couple of sets, where I couldn't get into the room on time. Like, I have to properly protect myself with like a mask and the gloves. But meanwhile, the patient is crashing. And I just can't get there on time. So, it's – she ended up dying … And I know it's like, it's not my fault. But it's the system – it makes it really difficult. And so, I like, I've gone into counselling, so I can just make sure I don't feel the guilt.

Nurses also felt guilty when they were unable to provide emotional care they recognized patients needed, particularly due to restrictions on visits from family and friends. While policies required nurses to reduce the time they spent with patients to diminish the chance of transmitting COVID-19, patients' need for emotional comfort increased.

This held true especially for nurses working with populations who had pre-existing needs for holistic care that could not be reconciled with pandemic protocols. Nurses expressed deep concern and "heart-break" for those who did not have access to safe spaces and those for whom physical distancing policies greatly increased their risk of violence or overdose. For these nurses and their clients, COVID-19 was layered onto pre-existing crises, such as the overdose crisis, increasing the trauma from all those crises and making them unbearable. One nurse explained that she was forced to take time off work following a debriefing with a client who had witnessed their boyfriend die of an overdose. The nurse described "heaviness in my chest. I went home and couldn't stop crying." Another nurse noted that while she had witnessed COVID-19-related deaths, overdoses and toxic drug deaths were also rising, and the combined traumas were leading to complex needs within the affected communities. She described clients calling to say they were suicidal: "This is not only a COVID problem, but mental health is a problem. People are depressed and choosing to kill themselves versus asking for help." In such instances, nurses felt responsible for these patients but could not help them stay safe, and experienced extreme second-hand trauma and grief.

Several participants explained that, within the preceding year, they had been diagnosed with major depression, anxiety, and/or PTSD for the first time in their lives. One nurse said, "I was diagnosed with severe depression, severe anxiety in the context of post-traumatic stress disorder. I have never had mental health issues in my entire life. I can actually talk about that today without crying, but seven months ago if you asked me how was work, I'd burst into tears and shut down." Many described the difficulties they had sleeping and/or eating as the physical manifestations of stress. The sources of poor mental health included both home and work responsibilities. On the one hand, it was difficult for nurses to focus at work due to the stress and anxiety they felt over their family's well-being. On the other hand, longer and more strenuous hours at work affected their family relationships because it limited the time they had to spend with their families and they were exhausted. In addition, as COVID-19 was constantly discussed in all facets of their lives, many felt overwhelmed, because they could never disconnect.

Several nurses turned to using substances such as alcohol, antidepressants, and over-the-counter medications as a method of coping. One nurse confessed, "It was the only way to shut my mind off. I got tired; I'd have a glass of wine and I'd be like 'OK now I can go to bed,' but ... my mind was just spinning, so Benadryl and wine, that was my cocktail." Another nurse reported using a similar "cocktail":

> As nurses, we're so good at compartmentalizing ... You see a lot
> of traumatic things, you sometimes are dealing with patients that
> are just in the aftermath of trauma and you got to put that in a
> box or in a room inside your mind and that's your work box,
> right? And when your home life is out of kilter and you don't have
> your support people, you don't have things to put back into your
> emotional bank, then you start to run on empty and then you take
> Benadryl and wine and hope that everything goes away.

Some nurses started or increased smoking. Others were taking prescription drugs such as sleeping, anti-anxiety, and antidepressant medication.

Nurses explained that staffing shortages prevented them from taking time for healthier forms of self-care. The extremely high workloads made it nearly impossible to decompress and process traumatic situations. A nurse who had witnessed a COVID-19-related death explained,

> Sometimes you go through second-hand grief almost, going
> through a difficult situation at work, and you feel really
> overwhelmed. But the department is busy, so you can't go
> for a walk for thirty minutes; you can't really decompress ...
> You're in a full assignment and doing things while your head
> is somewhere else, and you're just trying to function and do
> all the tasks and not make any mistakes.

Another noted that her request for a mental health day had been rejected due to a lack of staff to cover her shifts: "We have personal days we can take, and I've tried to take six and been denied those six just because we don't have staff coverage." Those who did manage to get time off described feeling guilty about calling in sick or taking a mental health day, feeling that a COVID-19-related absence was the only justifiable reason for missing work. Staffing shortages not only increased their stress and anxiety at work but also prevented nurses from taking measures to mitigate such threats to their mental health.

Nurses described previously dealing with workplace challenges through their peer support networks, but these were weakened by

COVID-19 physical distancing and colleagues' exhaustion from being overworked, restricting not only in-person interactions but also their individual capacity to support others. One nurse said that the inability to support each other "makes it like swimming in quicksand sometimes." Another noted that what "messes me up is seeing my colleagues in distress. I want to give more and more but physically and mentally just can't." Another noted that while the nurses did debrief cases with one another, it was always a neutral or professional experience. Lack of time and energy compounded by physical distancing inhibited nurses' ability to support one another.

A few nurses had either increased their counselling sessions or had begun therapy during the pandemic. One nurse described needing to go to therapy just to hear repeatedly that she was not a bad nurse and that she was not a bad person for smoking, after taking up the habit as a form of stress relief. However, most nurses did not access the mental health supports provided by their employers. This confirms previous research findings that most nurses do not access workplace mental health supports to deal with workplace stress (MacPhee, Dahinten, and Havaei 2017). One nurse explained that such approaches put the responsibility on the individual as opposed to recognizing that the causes of poor mental health were system-wide: "They keep sending you emails and 'By the way, look after your mental health, here's a link.' That's about the extent of it … You're not busy enough, you're not stressed enough. Here you go, you also need to manage your mental health better … It's on you." Nurses did not call phone numbers or access the websites provided because they did not have the time and because they recognized that such services would not address the root causes of their poor mental health – being overworked in a highly stressful environment and rarely being supported by their managers.

Nurses suggested improving mental health supports through an active rather than passive approach. One nurse explained, "[L]ike there's, it's definitely a passive kind of approach to mental health and I think that there needs to be a lot more done in terms of people coming in." Another nurse recommended, "I feel that if there was more check-ins and some sort of like mental health support where we felt like it's there, like we can go. It's not like calling these 1-800 numbers and talking to someone on the phone and having an inconsistency where it's kind of on you, versus like someone is just there." Sharing a positive example of helpful mental health support, another nurse noted that it "went a long way when a hospital psychiatrist gave everyone a pep talk that wasn't about protocols. It made people feel like someone was listening, especially because the psychiatrist also had young kids and understood the struggles nurses were experiencing."

A number of respondents either left work temporarily or were considering leaving the field due to the effects on their mental health. For example, three people on one participant's team went on leave following the first lockdown. She linked the attrition to the lack of pandemic preparedness and its effects on the nurses' mental health:

> We were not prepared. They all talked about "Oh, pandemic planning, we're all prepared from the start." No, we failed. We sucked. We did a horrible job, and the healthcare workers are going to pay for it mentally for many years after this. We even have nurses at stake ... There's a lot of people who are like, 'I'm only staying for my colleagues and as soon as this pandemic is over, I'm no longer going to be a nurse.'"

One nurse described taking a temporary leave and sleeping for three weeks straight because she was exhausted. Another noted that she was currently off work because she had had a nervous breakdown from trying to work from home, manage a caseload of thirty-nine acute clients over the phone, run groups over Zoom, and attend doctors' appointments with clients. Such accounts reflect the determinants behind survey findings in May 2021 that 35 per cent of nurses were considering leaving the profession (BCNU 2021) and previous research showing that burnout is a predictor of nurse turnover (Poghosyan, Aiken, and Sloane 2009). A nurse who had taken a medical leave for mental health reasons described "the immense guilt of having to make that choice to step away during a global pandemic and an opioid crisis, I think that guilt was the hardest. It absolutely killed me to make that choice. It was the hardest decision I ever made in my life, and I still regret it and feel immense guilt and shame that I couldn't do it despite doing the very best that I could." Many noted that it wasn't the work, which nurses previously got value from, causing them to leave the field, but the pace and the workload: "People are burnt out, but I'm not tired of nursing. I love nursing; I just think I'm overworked."

This love for nursing and commitment to patients and colleagues led many nurses to persevere. One nurse explained that despite diagnosing herself with depression, she continued to work, saying, "I was willing and able to go to work in that completely broken state because I'm a nurse and that's what nurses do." Another nurse described being "ready to quit and throw away [her] career" in July 2020, but then decided, "[N]o, I'm a nurse, I can do this. I just have to get myself healthy to get back on the boat." While such commitment is admirable and sustains the COVID-19 response, it is also exploitable, with potential long-term negative effects on nurses' health – particularly considering the high rates of PTSD reported – and therefore the resilience of the healthcare system.

POWER

Nurses felt that hospital decision-making prioritized scientific research, which was admittedly nascent and constantly changing during the initial months of the pandemic, over their knowledge as frontline responders. One nurse explained that she felt COVID-19-related decisions centred on "research says this, so the policy is this," as opposed to asking nurses what they knew on the basis of their lived experiences. Nurses felt that this focus limited the effectiveness of the response to COVID-19 and contributed to nurses feeling disempowered, with one explaining, "I would like to at least be involved. If they're going to implement a new change or policy, I would love for my opinion to be heard, or my thoughts, just because I think that a lot of the initiatives taken sometimes aren't taken from the frontline staff's considerations – like, how much time that adds to our day. Or how much that small change affects patient care or time management." Many nurses described never being asked by management for their input, while those who were asked often felt their insights weren't listened to: "It's almost like 'I'm asking because I've been told I have to ask you as an employee what you see or feel or want to do. But I'm going to do what we're going to do anyway.' That's basically it." Nurses often felt that nobody valued their expertise as frontline care providers who had intimate knowledge of the effects of these policies on patients and health systems.

Because of a lack of meaningful consultation, nurses did not trust those making decisions, seeing them as distanced from patient care: "When you're in that office space, I think a lot of people ... just don't know what nurses go through or what we're dealing with on a daily basis, and they kind of forget about, is this practical, is this going to even work? Is it even going to be implemented?" They commented on how many of those in decision-making roles worked from home or remote offices and had only second-hand knowledge of the day-to-day challenges nurses were facing and what policies were feasible. As a result, they felt that management did not recognize the multiple relationships between workload, pandemic uncertainty, mental health effects, and patient care. One nurse reflected on how the protocols and being exhausted limited her ability to provide care, something she felt the decision-makers didn't consider. "We are throwing ourselves in harm's way in order to make sure that that one person survives that event. I just feel like, if that was, you know, say a policymaker reading this, like if that was his brother, or his son, he would probably want to make sure that nurse is well-rested, fed … If they knew what it was like in our shoes to have to like – we're throwing ourselves into danger, but we're held back because we have to make sure we're protected." They identified a disconnect between designing protocols and implementing protocols, which they saw as resulting from management making decisions at a level removed from patient care and done without consulting nurses.

For example, many nurses did not have the power to determine and access the PPE they needed to protect themselves while providing care to patients. During the initial months of the pandemic, participants described sanitizing and recycling N95 masks to conserve them because the supply was limited, and reusing gloves and masks. A number of nurses felt other essential workers had greater protection than they did: "Our paramedics [are] in N95 masks … a shield, gloves up to here, a full suit, and we're running around with a little mask on our face. And the police, the same. They have filtered masks. And [we] are your healthcare providers. And so, I totally feel like our whole profession was disrespected." Lack of protection was a particular concern for immunocompromised or pregnant nurses. In some instances, employers only allowed access to PPE at designated times and under supervision: "The first thing that they did at my workplace was lock up all the PPE, so we didn't have access to masks right off the bat, even just plain masks or gowns or gloves … Twice a day the door would be unlocked for an hour, somebody stood in that room and watched us and counted each and every glove that we took." Nurses were often not told why protocols had changed, affecting their trust in those who were making the decisions. One nurse explained, "On some days we would have changes three, four times in one shift … If you were wearing an isolation gown to this room, the next day you weren't supposed to anymore, and then again you were. So, it just felt like, 'Wait, am I exposing myself?' Are the policies based on best practice, or are they based on supply and demand?" Nurses often felt that no one listened to their concerns when they expressed frustration with how PPE was allocated or suggested other arrangements. One nurse was told just to do her best when she brought up her concerns about regulations for masks not meeting standards. As a nurse, she felt she was required to take basic precautions and was uncomfortable doing what she felt compromised her patients' and colleagues' safety, but she had no recourse to challenge the directive.

When nurses were able to contribute to decision-making regarding the types of PPE to use, they felt better supported by the healthcare system. This also held when PPE was consistently available or when management explained any restrictions on its use and provided timelines on when new supplies would arrive. Open communication from management on PPE availability increased nurses' positive feelings of accountability and transparency from management. One participant described successfully advocating for higher-level PPE for nurses working with COVID patients. Another noted that when nurses with children or immunocompromised household members requested permission to wear N95s, management agreed, even though it was not hospital policy. Similarly, some nurses reported that management involved them in broader COVID-19-related decision-making and responded to their requests and concerns. In one instance, the leadership supported nurses' idea of creating a dedicated staff room for those providing COVID-19 care. In another, the manager would write down team concerns, bring them to the meeting, and come back with answers. Nurses in these contexts described meaningful consultation as being not only empowering but also increasing their sense of safety.

CONCLUSION

Expectations that nurses would work long hours with few breaks and fill unpaid care deficits at home, while dodging COVID infection and stigma, suggest that the assumption that nurses could battle numerous foes at once (like an invincible robot in a sci-fi movie) was prevalent. Such assumptions, strengthened by nurses' status as essential workers, forced them to keep working even when they were on the brink of burnout, despite having inconsistent access to necessities, including coffee, child care, and bathroom breaks. An unsustainable workload affected not only nurses' ability to provide the patient care they felt was required but also their ability to care for their own children and other dependents at home. One nurse reflected, in March 2021, "That's what it feels like, we lived through hell and survived, but barely." Since that interview, nurses have continued to survive and provide care to COVID-19 and other patients and to family members at home. This perseverance is impressive but that very dedication can lead to nurses suffering from PTSD, with long-term effects on their own well-being and that of the health system.

The nurses' experiences shared in this chapter demonstrate the need to reform the health system, including increasing and modifying strategies to better support nurses, during both normal circumstances and times of crises. Given their integral role during the pandemic, nurses' lived experience constitutes expertise that could inform systems and policies to strengthen pandemic preparedness and response. Participants shared key recommendations on where to start. These include creating family-friendly policies and work environments by providing on-site child care and improved access to child care in the community, allowing flexible work schedules, and offering paid care days. Nurses emphasized that PPE needs to be accessible, appropriate, and available, with nurses involved in the decisions made for PPE usage. Many noted the need to address the stigma around poor mental health and actively, rather than passively, provide mental health support, such as through on-site services. They further emphasized that access to fresh and healthy meals during their shifts would greatly increase their well-being. The pandemic has added urgency to previous calls to invest in training, hiring, and better working conditions for nurses to address persistent shortages. Nurses' service throughout the pandemic justifies greater investments in their well-being and personal and professional development.

5

Picking Up the Pieces

Moms

I'm a single mom. This is how I show up in the world, it's a huge part of how I identify. There's a lot of things that have to be done because there is no other choice. I have tiny humans to keep alive and try to keep their mental health ok through a pretty earth-shaking experience. I mean if nobody else is going to show up, you can pretty much count on the mom. She will show up and that is beautiful and wonderful, but also heavily fucking exploited.

Community health worker and mom

I'd been expecting the email from my kid's childcare centre. It was bound to come at some point, and there it was. The subject line read, "IMPORTANT COVID Exposure Information." The centre would earn the dubious distinction of having the largest childcare facility outbreak of COVID-19 in the province, which was eventually traced back to a super-spreader pub trivia night. It was so high-profile that the provincial government used it for an infographic (see figure 5.1).

While catchy, I felt the infographic was incomplete. It was missing a box that showed the number of parents (at least twenty) who had to take care of their COVID-19-positive children. It was also missing a box that showed the number of parents (over one hundred) who now had toddlers isolating at home because they were close contacts. But these secondary effects of COVID-19 don't lend themselves to infographics, so the work and the effects of parenting during a pandemic remain largely invisible. Like the women who saw their sons,

← **Thread**

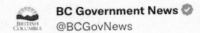

BC Government News ✓
@BCGovNews

It only takes one person and one night for COVID-19 to spread quickly. By limiting our social interactions and following public health restrictions, we can help keep our schools, daycares and communities safe. #CovidBC

From just one COVID-19 positive person at a pub trivia night...

28 people from the pub night tested positive, including 24 customers and 4 staff members

10 people tested positive for COVID-19 after close contact with someone from the pub trivia night (excludes daycare transmission)

2 daycare staff went to work after attending the pub trivia night, which resulted in transmissions to other people in the daycare

27 people tested positive as a result of transmission at the daycare

8 workplace exposures from people at the pub trivia night who went to work sick. This includes two industrial sites, two offices, a restaurant, and a store

1 school staff member tested positive after coming into contact with another school staff member who was at the pub trivia night, leading to an entire class having to self-isolate

15 additional people tested positive after close contact with people from the daycare

296 total people exposed to COVID-19 and required to self-isolate at home, unable to go to work or school

Based on data from Fraser Health, February 26, 2021.

COVID-19 IN BC

Figure 5.1 BC government infographic on outbreak in childcare facility

husbands, and brothers march off to the First and Second World Wars, and then quietly fought hunger, illness, and anxiety at home, parents' contributions occur behind closed doors.

In heterosexual parenting relationships in Canada, parenting labour is not shared equally. While men have taken on more parenting responsibilities over the past two decades, women still do the majority of childcare-related tasks, with one study showing that men did 38 per cent and women 62 per cent of childcare labour in 2015 (Guppy, Sakumoto, and Wilkes 2019). Gender roles in unpaid care in the home reflect long-standing gender inequities within Canada, such as a gender pay gap (16.5 per cent on average in 2020) and social norms about who is responsible for unpaid care work (Collins et al. 2020).

Even before the pandemic, these inequities were exacerbated by the lack of access to paid child care. A pre-COVID-19 study found that childcare fees in most cities were unaffordable. Another noted that 44 per cent of non-school-aged children lived in "childcare deserts" where there are not enough childcare spaces available to meet needs (Macdonald 2018). BC, in particular, has a legacy of high fees and few spaces. A 2018 survey found that 46.5 per cent of BC families with children under five had difficulty accessing child care (Edwards 2020). As noted in chapter 7, the childcare sector in the province has been described as chaotic and unorganized because of a mix of provider types (for-profit and not-for-profit, institutional and home-based, licensed and unlicensed); varying working conditions for educators; and a lack of accessibility for parents (Milne 2016). Lack of accessible child care influences mothers' decisions to delay returning to the workforce more often than fathers' following parental leave, and to take on part-time instead of full-time work, which affects their financial security and career development, and exacerbates the motherhood penalty (the difference in earnings between women who have children and those who do not) perpetuated by societal norms and discriminatory hiring practices.

What childcare options existed for parents were extinguished in March 2020 when a public health emergency was declared across the country, schools and childcare centres were closed, and provisions were made only for the children of essential workers. Suddenly, the 700,000 children under fourteen in BC were stuck at home, and someone had to make sure they were safe, educated, fed, and cared for. While schools reopened in June, and most child care also subsequently opened, education and care continued to be interrupted throughout the first year of the pandemic (and beyond) as children with symptoms were told to stay home until their symptoms resolved and those designated a close contact were told to isolate for a minimum of ten days. In addition to increased physical care needs, children and youth required emotional support as their routines and sense of normalcy were repeatedly disrupted. The task of mothering – in the amount of time needed to commit to it and in its complexity – became greater.

The Canadian federal government responded to the needs of families primarily through cash transfers during the initial months of COVID-19. In May 2020, parents benefited from a one-time increase in the Canada child benefit of $300 extra per child. This was in addition to CERB, which provided $2,000 per month to those who lost work due to COVID-19 and met the eligibility requirements. Similarly, the Province of BC provided one-time payments, such as the BC emergency benefit for workers, of $1,000 to those receiving CERB. As this chapter will illustrate, while these payments provided financial relief, they did not address the increased care burdens placed on women's shoulders by gender norms and economic structures, the heightened risk of violence against women and children, or the resulting stress and anxiety.

The experiences in this chapter come from a range of mothers interviewed during the first year of the pandemic (March 2020 to March 2021). While many of the women in the other chapters are also mothers, and their mothering experiences are discussed in sections on the quadruple burden, this chapter flips the narrative and focuses solely on the work of mothering and how it interacts with women's other roles. The twenty-three mothers whose experiences are included here range from those with secure employment living in upper-middle-class neighbourhoods to those who are unemployed and living in transition housing. The number of children within these families ranges from one to four. Eight mothers are newcomers to Canada, and there is a specific focus on their experiences and those of single mothers (seven women) and mothers of children with special needs (five women). In addition, I spoke to four key informants from organizations that provide services to women and children to develop a deeper understanding of the broader context. As in the other chapters, the experiences here are not meant to be generalizable or representative. Instead, I aim to share these mothers' experiences as one window into the multiple effects of COVID-19 on women, their children, and their families.

THE QUADRUPLE BURDEN

During the initial months of the pandemic, women represented 58 per cent of those forced out of work, despite making up only 45 per cent of the Canadian workforce. Feminized industries, such as food service and tourism, experienced COVID-19-related closures, and many women left the workforce to care for their children because of school and childcare interruptions (Shrma and Smith 2021). One mother explained, "In February my contract was renewed for the year until December of this year and then as COVID-19 hit and air travel, as you can imagine, just jumped off a cliff so they had to cancel my contract. Since then, I have not been able to find work." Caregiving responsibilities caused gender employment gaps to widen among parents of young children between February and May 2020 (Qian and Fuller 2020). In dual-income-earning households, decisions about who would give up work were often determined by the gender wage gap; as one mother explained, "And I just thought, well I guess you [her husband] make more so I guess I'm the one staying home." In April 2020, mothers between the ages of twenty-four and fifty-five lost 26 per cent of their work hours for family and health reasons compared with 14 per cent for fathers (BCWHF 2020). Another mother described being forced to reduce her paid work because of the lack of child care: "I mean the biggest thing at the very beginning for myself was my child care for my dependents. I actually had to take … 50 per cent of my job off to care for them because, at least in our community, there is an absolute childcare crisis already. And COVID made that so much worse." Those who were forced to leave work, whether due to sector or childcare impacts, were concerned about their ability to return to work, largely due to the continued uncertainty about child care, with one mother noting, "[R]egarding work, I'm not sure if I can return to work, because there's no daycare or preschool for my children." Lack of child care further inhibited their ability to find new job opportunities. A single mother reflected that she had tried to do a phone interview with her two small children at home: "I had one phone call about a job application and the HR person asked how I would manage with the kids at home. I did not hear back." Such experiences shed light on statistics that show it took women twice as long (thirteen months) as men to find work, compared with pre-lockdown levels (Shrma and Smith 2021).

Even once childcare centres reopened, high fees created a further barrier to returning to work, particularly for women financially affected by the pandemic. The mother quoted above, who lost work due to the decline in tourism, explained, "And also economically I just felt like you know having to pay $2,000 a month I just really couldn't afford it especially because my contract was cancelled." In this case, the approximately $2,000 in childcare fees was equal to the amount provided by the Canadian government through CERB. Even those who were continuing to work were concerned about the cost, particularly in light of the risk of further interruptions in care as childcare centres told them that symptomatic children would have to stay home: "Like it's expensive, so if we do decide to go, I mean, kids pick up stuff from each other so quickly that all of a sudden we could be like a week in and then we have to be out for two weeks ... well, the likelihood is pretty high and then we're out half the money of daycare for the month." Such concerns may partly explain subsequent trends, across the country, of declining childcare enrolments in 2020 (Macdonald and Friendly 2021).

Lack of child care further exacerbated the pre-existing motherhood penalty by interrupting career advancement and educational opportunities. A mom described receiving "threats from my employer that if I didn't get back to work, then what? Not an overt threat, but there was always the threat of 'You need to get back to work and figure this out.' I felt like I was drowning every single day." Another mother's education had been interrupted, inhibiting her career advancement, "and then the daycare closed so I couldn't finish my practicum anyway ... I was kind of upset because it was like I don't have child care and I can't, I can't finish." Similarly, mothers who had recently immigrated to Canada noted that they were unable to continue with language classes essential for career development, which had moved online, because their children, now at home, constantly interrupted their learning. This suggests that the COVID penalty for women will adversely affect their long-term career advancement and income.

To meet their financial needs, mothers who had lost work applied for CERB and related programs, which they described as "quite a lifesaver." Others were able to access student benefits, and many noted that the increase in the federal child benefit helped them meet COVID-19-related gaps in their income. However, a number of single mothers reflected that while the CERB money was welcome, they still struggled to access food and PPE, particularly during lockdown, when many necessities were scarce and there were lineups at many shops. One respondent explained: "My fear was I don't have food for my son in the fridge. That was my biggest fear because I know I have money in my bank account, but there is nothing in the store and I feel like I'm supposed to not take my son ... I went to get groceries; it was a long line – my son doesn't have – like he doesn't want to be standing." Without child care and unable to rely on external support networks, single mothers spoke of the challenges of having to take children with them to visit multiple shops, often via public transit, which increased their risk of COVID-19 exposure, to find necessities: "I sometimes have to make two trips because kids lose patience. I went out today and turned around because I knew the kids wouldn't make it [standing in line]. It is hard to find hand sanitizer. I wish I could find masks for kids." Similarly, another single mother described the anxiety and guilt she experienced every time she needed to get groceries:

I asked my neighbour, "Can you look after my son, I need to go for milk and eggs, and I don't want to bring my son there," and she said, "Sorry, I can't." ... And then I just took my son with me, and I go to the cashier who was like, "Why are you taking your kid to get groceries," and I was just, "I don't know where to put him," like I can't leave him alone, right? ... I feel like I was being a very bad mom.

Respondents reported going without fresh fruit and vegetables, eggs, and milk. Others noted that the amount provided by CERB was insufficient considering the costs of living in BC's Lower Mainland, where a livable wage was considered about \$2,800 per month (Ivanova 2022). A newcomer mother of three, who had lost her food sector job, explained that her rent alone was \$2,200, \$200 more than CERB.

Some mothers were unable to access CERB and related income supports. Two single mothers had lost work a week before CERB was implemented and had already applied for EI (Employment Insurance), which made them ineligible for CERB. As a result, one was receiving \$400 and the other \$1,200 per month, compared with the \$2,000 provided by CERB. Those who lost work hours but not their jobs were often unable to apply for CERB, because it was only provided to those earning less than \$1,000 per month. The mother who could not find alternative child care so switched to part-time work noted, "I lost 50 per cent of my income but I was like one hour under the threshold for CERB.

So, I went for three or four months with a very, very tight budget for my family." A newcomer mother explained that she continued a part-time job as a physiotherapist because she did not want to lose the chance to build her Canadian experience: "I work in two centres. One of them doesn't need me right now because of the decrease of clients, you know. But another one calls me. I can start one day a week, hopefully, if they have work and I am because I am on subcontract, not employee. So, if they have cases, clients, they give me clients ... And still if they don't have enough clients, I don't have job." Not only did her work prevent her from accessing CERB, but the precarious conditions caused her a high degree of financial uncertainty and stress.

On 15 March 2020, the federal government put out a work-from-home advisory. At that time, more women than men in Canada were working in positions that enabled them to work from home (Statistics Canada 2020a), but this did not necessarily make balancing care and work commitments possible. As pre-COVID-19 research has shown, working from home can cause a blurring of boundaries and heightened levels of stress (Hjálmsdóttir, Bjarnadóttir, and Eðvarðs Sigurðssonar 2021). Such challenges became even more acute when children were no longer in child care or school during working hours. For single mothers without child care, the expectation that they would work from home seemed like a joke. One reflected, "When something like this happens and we were asked to work from home, and also care for our kids at the same time, it's kind of like we understand that's two jobs, but yet the system doesn't recognize it's two jobs and there's no consideration made around it to make sure that we're managing two jobs, right? It's never – somehow, it's just like yeah, the kids are home, yay, you're good to go. No." She described trying to continue to conduct scientific research with her two-year-old on her lap.

Many noted that it was mothers, rather than fathers, who were expected to manage such impossible tasks. A mother who was separated from her child's father explained that she took on childcare responsibilities when centres and schools closed because the father "doesn't think it's his realm." Even in families where both partners could work from home, mothers noted that in most instances, they were expected to manage child care. One partnered mother noted, "I became, you know, the person responsible for the kids 24/7 and it sort of became obvious that I'm the person responsible for the kids. I mean, we both need child care to work, right, my husband also needs child-care, he wants to go to work, but I don't think he really gets that. It's obvious somebody's going to take care of the kids. He doesn't have to do anything." Others recognized that they took on childcare responsibilities "almost voluntarily, you know. Because we feel that responsibility." Women's remarks on how quickly they fell into the primary parenting role reflect a similar realization to those recorded in a study from Iceland, a country consistently ranked as the highest in gender equality. The study found that women "seemed to be stunned by how uneven the division of labor turned out to be during the pandemic" (Hjálmsdóttir, Bjarnadóttir, and Eðvarðs Sigurðssonar 2021). Gender norms were exacerbated in the exceptional circumstances of the pandemic.

As a result, women's paid work suffered. The single mom who tried to conduct research with her two-year-old on her lap said, "My work productivity is probably, you know, about 40 per cent less than what it usually was." A mother who also employed other women noted, "When I look at our employees, women are still the ones who are primarily responsible for their children and for their households. We still have that gender difference, and there's still the pressure for them to be at work ... So, the impact on mental health and stability of the family, I think, is going to be an ongoing issue." While the Canada Labour Code was amended to provide for absences for reasons related to COVID-19, and BC instituted three days of unpaid job-protected leave, these actions did not extend to unprecedented childcare responsibilities. As a result, moms were expected to work from home despite childcare interruptions – often an impossible task that necessarily interrupted their productivity, potentially further negatively affecting their career and income-earning opportunities into the future.

Women further argued that care work included more than just doing the physical care, but they had a hard time articulating the triple burden they carried:

> It could be that it's my imagination. It's not just the physical, you know, taking care of them ... there's this whole other layer of, it's not exactly work, and you can't really quantify it but you're doing it all the time. Like oh how do I make sure that they still keep in touch with their friends, how do I make sure that they have the clothes that they need because, you know, nothing is open. They're still eating normal food and they're keeping a routine, like all those things that it's sort of a, it's all my mind, mind work.

The mental load of managing families and households, which women predominantly bear in non-crisis times as well as during crises, was exacerbated in a context of uncertainty and increased needs (McLaren et al. 2020). Another mother noted, "And, like I said, there's lots of lack of clarity around exactly what is happening. So, and I'm sort of the one that kind of ends up managing it because my husband has to deal with his job and anything that's around that, but everything else is my, my thing." Everything else included trying to ensure their children's mental health, calling relatives and friends to check in, and keeping up to date on the most recent COVID-19 guidelines. Pandemic uncertainty and the lack of paid care increased not only women's physical and custodial care work but also the even less visible mental load.

Alongside providing unpaid care, mothers were often responsible for online learning as schooling went virtual. A mother who did shift work noted, "[W]e were homeschooling two children and we also had a third one at home, so I ended up having to cancel a lot of work, so I think there was some internal struggle there." While homeschooling posed challenges for all parents, single-parent families and households with fewer resources were particularly affected by the digital divide. Single mothers described sharing their cell phones – the only digital devices in the house – with their children for online learning, which they recognized was inadequate. Others described trying to arrange for their two children to share one computer or tablet, which was impossible when their classes were scheduled at the same time. A newcomer mother explained, "We actually realized that we didn't have the right technology to do the online learning. We discovered that we can't use an iPad – the iPad does not work for it, just because of the interface ... And then we had a laptop, a different laptop, and they were, like, it's too slow, it's too slow." Other newcomer mothers explained the challenge of trying to help their children with schoolwork that they were unfamiliar with. One woman commented, "I don't know this language. I don't know this type of math. How do I help my son? I worry he will fall behind." Some community organizations and school districts provided families in need with laptops and related supports, but there were often long waiting lists because supplies were inadequate.

Newcomers, who relied on community services for recreation and to overcome educational inequities, were further affected. A newcomer mother who had lost work due to COVID-19 said,

We just pay for basic needs, not for extra … For instance,
I think my daughter ask me I want to have – I want to order
this book. She find it online and I explain for her I couldn't pay
lots of money for book, for buying book, and she not believing
and before COVID we borrow at library … I think everywhere
were closed and she told me I read some of them twice or
three times. It's boring. I need more books.

Another newcomer mother worried about how her children
would be able to develop their English language skills and socialize
without education programs.

In such instances, moms felt guilty for not being able to meet their
children's educational and development needs. One mom explained,
"I've felt really like poor mom because at the beginning I still had
work to do. Especially like when I had meetings and stuff was for him
to just watch shows, or a TV, or electronics. I really don't like him
being in front of it so I feel really badly about it, but it was very challenging." Another mother explained, "I think from a development
standpoint like that mom guilt that you know, your child's getting –
I mean some days – my Fridays for instance. I have meetings that …
start at 8:00 in the morning and run until midday before I get a
break … I feel like sometimes I'm throwing snacks at her as she walks
past me. And the TV is on." While recognizing that COVID-19
increased their workload in both paid and unpaid work, women still
felt guilty for cutting corners, particularly for child care. Guilt over
their inability to manage an increasing number of tasks is a persistent
feature of motherhood in Canadian society, rooted in patriarchal
cultural and labour norms (Watson 2020). That such harmful gender
norms persisted even in the exceptional context of COVID-19 only
demonstrates how deeply rooted they are.

BEING ESSENTIAL

As described above, the work of mothering is essential to children's
well-being, development, and education, with moms feeling immense
guilt when they could not fulfill their own expectations. However, no
list of essential workers includes parents, which means they did not
receive PPE, pandemic pay (or pay at all), COVID-19-related sick
leave, access to counselling, or other services provided to essential
workers. While most parents struggled to some degree as a result,

mothers of children with special needs in particular found that essential services for their children were stripped away, with responsibility instead placed on their shoulders.

During the initial months of the pandemic, when schools and child-care centres closed, supports that had been in place for children with special needs and their families, such as behavioural interventions and counselling, were abruptly halted. One mom explained the effect of school closures on her family: "Supports for special-needs children went away overnight with COVID. The school didn't step up even though the government said kids were supposed to be supported and that they would have daycare options. The supports didn't exist because they are special needs. Schools stalled and stalled. It was devastating, unbelievably frustrating." She advocated on behalf of her kids to the superintendent of schools, and the school opened up space to children with special needs, but only for respite care, not education, because the teaching assistants had been laid off and the teachers were working from home, providing online education to the other students. The mom reflected on how she had put in a sustained effort to ensure that her children had the services they needed, which was then negated: "I built this empire around my kids and this whole structure and it just like disappeared overnight and then the government just wasn't there. And they, I just, there were so many [parents]. I mean they were just flabbergasted. There was nothing. Like how were these support people not essential workers?" The mother, an essential worker herself, asked, "How am I supposed to work and be essential and help if I don't have that support for my children? ... I've had to rework my entire life to meet their needs." As a result, she was left juggling her essential role as a mother with her essential role as a healthcare provider.

Interruptions to services in schools and childcare settings adversely affected the well-being of children with special needs, which in turn affected the unpaid care work and well-being of mothers. A single mother described her child suffering severe anxiety due to the family's past experience of violence. Having fled the violent situation, the family had recently had to move to a crowded and noisy part of the city, where it was also hard for her child to sleep. The child had been receiving therapy at their childcare centre, but that ended abruptly with COVID-19 closures. The transition of moving, combined with his child care closing and his therapy then being interrupted, was taking a severe toll on the child's health. The previous night, he had gotten so anxious that he had started vomiting. The mother had called the nurses' hotline, which advised her to keep the child home and comfortable due to the perceived risk of COVID if she went to the hospital. A newcomer mother similarly noted that the closure of child care had exacerbated her daughter's anxiety, the result of fleeing conflict in Afghanistan, and had inhibited the daughter's progress in learning English. She worried, "Before, my daughter wouldn't speak to any adults. She was just starting to say English words when the centre closed. Now she just hides and points again." Witnessing such regressions was devastating to mothers, who felt helpless in the face of their children's suffering.

These experiences converge with those in chapters 3 and 7 to confirm just how essential child care and schooling are, not only in providing education to children but also a safe space and other essential services, particularly for those most in need. When these essential services were abruptly terminated, the responsibility was shifted onto mothers, who often, while perpetually willing to sacrifice their time and well-being for their children, did not have the medical or educational expertise to meet their children's needs. So they were set up to fail at the job most important to them.

MENTAL HEALTH, MORAL DISTRESS, AND BURNOUT

A study conducted in June 2020, three months into the pandemic, found that 71 per cent of women in Canada were feeling more anxious, depressed, isolated, overworked, or ill because of the increased unpaid care work caused by COVID-19 they had to do (Oxfam Canada 2020). In April 2021, one year into the pandemic, a Canadian Women's Foundation poll found that almost half of mothers were "reaching their breaking point." Further research found a cyclical relationship between child and maternal mental health, with concern over their children's mental health a top source of poor mental health among parents (Gadermann et al. 2021). Additional sources of stress related to moms' inability to manage both paid work and unpaid care burdens. As one mom explained, "[A]s a woman, as a mom, it's us that feel that you always need to be there to pick up the pieces."

Faced with multiple sources of stress, moms rarely had the time, privacy, or resources to access support. While the province had invested in virtual mental health supports early in the pandemic, most moms were not able to use them because, with their children constantly at home, they had no privacy. Also, according to a service provider, many of her clients lacked access to the technology and space needed to take advantage of virtual services: "[T]he ones who are impacted are those who don't have the privacy in their home to be able to resume the counselling, or the women who live in collective housing and don't have the technology or the privacy – and some women just don't – or they need the physical connection to be able to open up." A mother who had left a violent relationship had to discontinue her long-standing counselling after she lost her job and, therefore, her extended benefits, and she could not find a suitable replacement among the available free programs.

> From about a month before my separation up until February
> I was seeing a counsellor, a therapist on a pretty regular basis.
> But because of COVID-19, and because of the fact that I've now
> lost my job I don't really have health benefits, everything that,
> like counselling and things like that I have to pay out of pocket.
> I couldn't afford it, so I've kind of stopped that. She sent a list
> of resources that are supposed to be like free counselling but to
> be perfectly honest when I read through that list, I felt like none
> of it really applies, or nothing that I'm able to utilize.

Implementing virtual care through health authorities also meant that clients had to provide a provincial health card. This excluded those without immigration status. A newcomer mom who provided support to others noted, "It was quite hard for mums without status to be able to access online ... when these services closed down, when drop-in centres closed down, they didn't have any support available to them." Previously, many newcomer women had accessed services through community-based organizations, but these were now closed by public health orders.

Moms noted that they also had little time for self-care. A single mom noted, "I'm staying up later than I normally would just because I think that you know, by the end of the day I'm just – I just crave so much time to just do things for me." Another mom noted that she no longer had time to engage with a peer support group because with a child at home, she had no privacy, and asked, "[W]hen are we actually going to talk about our pain and suffering, when our kids are not around to listen?" Ironically, moms often felt guilty for their lack of self-care, saying they knew they should take care of themselves, but organizing self-care took mental labour they did not have the energy for, even if they had the time. Others questioned the discourse around self-care, with one mom demanding, "People need to stop telling me to do self-care and take care of myself because I don't have the frigging time to take care of myself and taking a bath is not going to cure the pandemic." The combination of high levels of stress and lack of time for self-care has the potential to lead to long-term negative health effects for mothers.

POWER

Much has been written about the rise of intimate partner violence (IPV) during the initial COVID-19 lockdown and the subsequent months (Kofman and Garfin 2020). In Canada, as in many contexts, the incidence and severity of IPV increased during the first year of COVID-19 due to stressors such as income loss or precarious employment, service disruptions, and lockdown measures (Yakubovich and Maki 2021). Researching IPV is ethically and methodologically complicated: it often results in low estimates of how often it is happening, relies on proxy indicators (such as calls to hotlines), and can retraumatize survivors (Lokot et al. 2021). For these reasons, during interviews or focus groups with mothers, I did not ask about their experiences of violence.

However, a number of women spoke voluntarily about feeling insecure or at increased risk of violence. Two single mothers noted that they were currently living in transition housing, and a third noted that she had recently separated from a violent partner. All three mentioned that COVID-19-related interruptions to child care had led to conflict with their children's other parent, because new shared care agreements had to be negotiated. One mother explained that her child's father did not understand that childcare centres were only open for essential workers and got angry with her when she asked him to share the increased childcare burden: "He just went ballistic. He just said that it's fine because they have not shut down daycares and he should be able to go to daycare … it's one of those combative issues that we just can't talk about." Another noted that her son's father disputed her decision to return their son to child care in June: "He's claiming that he didn't consent to our son going to this daycare even though he's been going there since he was fifteen months old."

Childcare interruptions also resulted in increased in-person contact with past partners. For some, that meant increased insecurity. A single mother explained,

> We did a lot of the exchanges with my son through daycare. There was a case of domestic violence which caused our separation. For me, it's very triggering to be close to, in the proximity of my ex. And because of the fact that [my son's] not going to daycare anymore we have to do the exchanges in person … I take my phone and I video-record it in a very obvious way. We've made the exchanges outside of [a grocery store] which luckily is always quite crowded. There's lots of people around and that makes me feel safer.

Childcare responsibilities are one of the most common points of tension within co-parenting relationships, and childcare interruptions caused by COVID-19 added to other pandemic stressors and increased points of conflict between parents, potentially exacerbating women's risk of violence (Silverio-Murillo, Balmori de la Miyar, and Hoehn-Velasco 2020).

The closure of family courts from March to July 2020 due to COVID-19 physical distancing policies also increased single mothers' sense of insecurity and risk of conflict with co-parents. While some court proceedings continued by teleconference, these were only for the most urgent cases, and usually pertained to child, not parent, safety. The postponement of all other cases exacerbated an already bad situation; family court cases can take years to resolve, with delays increasing the risk of future violence (Hrymak and Hawkins 2021). The mother quoted above, who had experienced IPV, explained how COVID-19 had affected her case:

> We were actually supposed to go to court in May, but because of COVID-19, they cancelled all the court proceedings and essentially, it's only in emergency situation[s] where they would hear any cases. Things kind of are in limbo right now. It's custody, it's a whole slew of things because if I say black, he'll say white. It just drags things on even longer, and already before COVID-19 it was extremely difficult in order to get a court date because of the fact that we have a long list of issues that we need to go through. We actually need like an all-day

hearing. And so, this was like in February or March that we got something for the end of May because it's just so difficult. Between like the court schedule of being able to get a court date and then also my ex's counsel, it's extremely difficult to get on her schedule. It was already difficult, and now with the whole COVID-19 thing, the courts are still not open and I'm not sure when they will be open. It's just – it's making things I think even worse.

Court proceedings exact a high emotional and financial toll on those leaving violent relationships (Vollans 2010), and COVID-19-related delays and changes to childcare arrangements increased and prolonged that toll.

Two mothers were unable to enforce child support payments from the other parent due to lack of access to family courts at this time, leading to renewed conflict. Refusing or delaying child support payments not only imposes financial hardship on mothers but can also be a form of abuse, continuing to draw out conflict and negatively affecting the other parent's well-being (Vollans 2010). One mother explained that her child's father was "taking advantage of this situation, and I can't go back to court because I have no money for a lawyer. I'm just trying to figure out how to get child support." This mother had already used the allocated number of hours provided by a legal aid retainer and no longer had access to representation, even if the courts had been functioning. As a result, she faced a double financial hit – losing both her job and her child support payments – alongside an escalated conflict with her child's other parent. COVID-19 court and childcare closures increased women's risk of conflict with co-parents, potentially contributing to IPV trends and financial and personal hardship.

CONCLUSION

When schools, child care, and community services closed, moms filled the gap. They provided the most essential work of keeping children safe, fed, and educated. Because moms already do this work on a regular basis, this contribution, while increasing dramatically, was rarely recognized, and it was never mentioned in discussions of essential work during the pandemic. No one clapped, banged pots, or offered free food and discounts to moms. Instead, increased unpaid care work was downloaded onto moms, who often blamed themselves when they could not meet the increasingly impossible demands.

Few policy responses to COVID-19 considered unpaid care burdens, and none explicitly recognized the gendered dimensions of care work. In contrast, mothers described unpaid care work as deeply gendered, disproportionately affecting women's economic security, career development, and overall well-being. Policy responses focused on providing financial support rather than accessible services and had a limited effect on access to care, or the well-being of care providers and their dependents. In particular, mothers of children with special needs struggled to provide the essential services their children required, with both mom and child suffering due to the impossibility of the task. Lack of access to child care further increased women's and children's insecurity, when the stress of making new arrangements and increased contact with co-parents heightened opportunities for conflict in the context of reduced access to justice. It is no wonder that so many mothers reported being on the verge of burnout a year into the pandemic. The long-term effects of carrying an impossible care burden for over two years can only be predicted, but current and past research suggests an increased risk of ongoing mental and physical health challenges, combined with a COVID-motherhood career penalty – both of which may exacerbate the other.

To mitigate both short- and long-term care burdens, mothers provided ideas on how future pandemic responses might offer greater support. One mom suggested that the negative effects of lockdown responses could be mitigated by providing necessities such as PPE and healthy food at central neighbourhood locations, such as schools and libraries. Another advocated for open-air drop-in childcare centres, such as on school grounds, for parents who need time to look for work or for self-care. Some mothers also noted that legal aid services needed to be increased, not decreased, during crises, and ensuring the continued operation of justice systems should be considered essential. On a more long-term and systems level, mothers suggested offering mental health support to parents at childcare centres, increasing access to affordable housing, and focusing on preventing, as opposed to just responding to IPV.

6

Nobody Wants to Be a Hero

Midwives

[In the] elevators to the perinatal unit was this superman figure
starting to rip open his shirt with hairy man hands ... I really did not
identify with that ... I don't feel like anyone knows I'm here and what
I do here ... Nobody wants to be a hero. Nobody wants to be working
in a pandemic. And that's not the acknowledgment that I want. I just
want the basic stuff.

Midwife

Midwives in BC have always had to be something of a revolutionary
force. For decades, Indigenous women, lay midwives, nurses, and others
in the women's health movement have advocated for pregnant people's
right to choose where, how, and under what conditions they would
receive maternity care (Benoit et al. 2005). In doing so, they have coun-
tered the historical shift from birth being treated as a natural event
cared for by midwives in the community to a medical pathology treated
by physicians in male-led facilities (Monteblanco 2021). By proving
the benefits and safety of midwifery care, midwives eventually achieved
status as an allied health profession within the BC health system
in 1998. The profession is now regulated by the BC College of Nurses
and Midwives, which requires all midwives to have a university degree
in midwifery or a related program.

   In 2020, there were about 300 midwives in BC (all women or gender-
diverse) providing publicly funded care to about 25 per cent of pregnant
people in the province each year (MABC 2022). Midwifery care differs

from that provided by medical doctors in that it is relationship-based and emphasizes prioritizing pregnant people's autonomy, dignity, and informed choice, including the option of a hospital or home birth. The Midwives Association of BC (MABC) describes its philosophy of care as based on "continuity of care, informed choice, choice of birth setting and collaboration with other health professionals." Appointments with midwives can last up to an hour, in contrast to doctors' appointments, which usually last less than fifteen minutes, with midwives providing whole-of-person care, including mental and emotional support. Midwife care during hospital delivery includes working closely with nurses and obstetricians, with most midwives also providing the option of home birth when it's safe to do so. Midwives visit new parents and their infants at home for the first month after birth, rather than asking them to come to a clinic, and they often offer postpartum support groups, physiotherapy, and counselling alongside medical care. Midwifery care is associated with fewer unnecessary medical interventions, cost savings to families and healthcare systems, higher rates of satisfaction with care, and autonomy around birth choices for pregnant people (Sandall et al. 2016). Demand for midwifery care in BC has grown over the past decade, outpacing the supply of midwives in many communities.

Despite the rapid growth of the profession, midwives, similar to physiotherapists, have been positioned as allied healthcare workers. That continues to situate them on the periphery of the health system, despite their close working relationships with other medical profession-als such as nurses and obstetricians. In BC, midwives are currently excluded from accessing the provincial benefits offered to other health-care workers, such as health and disability benefits, pensions, and parental and sick leave. They are paid substantially less for providing the same pre- and postnatal services as family physicians despite also having to cover costs for medical supplies and office overhead. In 2019, 34.7 per cent of midwives surveyed were considering leaving the pro-fession due to unsustainable workloads, the lack of benefits and job security, and the resultant burnout (Stoll and Gallagher 2019). The same year, the MABC rejected a contract proposed by the BC govern-ment on the basis of differences over wages and benefits, with negotiations going to arbitration (where they remain at the time of writing). It was in this context of already high rates of burnout and precarious work that midwives entered the pandemic, which further increased demand for their services, because many pregnant people saw home births as a way to reduce the risk of infection (Rudrum 2021).

To understand midwives' experiences during the COVID-19 pandemic, I held three focus groups and conducted four semi-structured interviews with a total of thirteen midwives between December 2020 and February 2021. Participants' experiences and perspectives reflect how this almost completely women-dominated sector, positioned at the margins of the health system and focused on maternal care, was made even more precarious by the pandemic, with potentially severe implications for midwives, parents, and infants.

THE QUADRUPLE BURDEN

During the initial months of the COVID-19 pandemic, demand for midwifery services increased, and midwives felt compelled to respond to parents' needs. One midwife explained, "Women deserve options in care and if we don't support a midwifery profession that's sustainable, child-bearing people will have less choice, and that will cause worse care to exist. Because when we don't have the balance of different care providers coming from different perspectives, women are offered less choices." Still, midwives could only take on so many clients, with one clinic noting that its waitlist grew to sixteen expectant parents during the first year of the pandemic, the highest it had ever been. COVID-19 also dramatically increased midwives' workload because they had to introduce new cleaning policies in their clinics, adapt to virtual care requirements, source PPE, and cover for each other following potential exposures or if someone was symptomatic. Midwives described working an additional twenty hours a week just trying to stay up to date with the most recent research on and public health guidance for COVID-19 and pregnancy. Many noted that the shift to virtual care and spaced in-person visits heightened expectant parents' anxiety, resulting in increased work following up by email and phone. Such emotional labour added to the already substantial time midwives dedicated to caring tasks, such as having longer appointments with expectant and new parents, providing emotional support and home visits or, as one midwife put it, "the care work that is typically unseen and uncompensated."

Increased midwifery work reduced the time midwives had for dependents at home. A midwife explained, "I'm spending more time away from my kids because it takes time to don and doff, and clean, and spread out your appointments, and do all the things that you need to do, so you're just pulled away so much more than you would like."

Less time with family heightened concerns about their children's well-being during the pandemic.

> The kids are miserable because they can't have play dates right now, so you always feel guilty, especially at the beginning of the pandemic when there was no school ... But even now you're constantly feeling guilty because they don't have friends to play with, they're missing school, you should be doing reading with them, you should play with them because they're upset too over COVID, and you just can't, like it's just not possible to do it all.

Because of the unpredictable hours of their work, many midwives had previously relied on relatives or nannies to care for their children. COVID-19 caused interruptions in both types of care. Many midwives chose to avoid contact with their children's grandparents for fear of passing on COVID-19 to them, and other care providers often chose to restrict their own bubbles. One midwife explained:

> Initially back in March and April, I remember thinking like, "Oh, this hasn't really affected my life too much." However, we had a nanny at that point, but then COVID got more intense, and she had to make choices of who's going to be in her bubble, and she had at-risk family members, and so then we lost our incredible nanny. And so being an on-call midwife business owner – my partner and I actually own the clinic together – we had basically no child care and we're just juggling back and forth.

In such situations, midwives described finding alternative child care as "virtually impossible" because of the lack of facilities providing care that corresponded to the hours of shift work. Another midwife recounted, "I have a six- and nine-year-old, and it's been brutal because like this is our first year without an official nanny, but we had like babysitters lined up for after school and stuff like that. But then they change, things change with COVID, they don't feel comfortable – it's the constant juggle." This constant juggling of increased midwifery workload in the context of reduced childcare support was overwhelming and exhausting, and midwives described the layered guilt they felt, that they were unable to do enough for their children, clients, and colleagues.

Midwives described their profession as "a lifestyle that the whole family adapts to" and "a blend between personal life and practice." The shift work and unpredictable hours meant that often a co-parent could take on much of the care work. As a result, many midwives who participated in this research were the main income earners in their families, heightening the financial risk associated with COVID-19. Several midwives had to take time off from work due to suspected or confirmed COVID-19 diagnoses, but as either the owners or staff of small practices, they did not have access to paid sick days. A midwife spoke of the challenge of balancing the need to isolate because of a COVID-19 exposure with the financial necessity of continuing to work: "My greatest stress about catching COVID is financial because my husband is unemployed, and if I get COVID and have to be off, even for two weeks, even if I have a mild form, that will affect us. And if I have to be off for a month, we won't be able to pay our mortgage." In August 2020, WorkSafeBC, the organization providing benefits to injured workers in BC, labelled COVID-19 an occupational risk illness, enabling workers quick access to coverage after exposure. However, midwives recounted that they had to put in substantial effort to prove they had contracted COVID-19 at work before they were able to access benefits, even after working with confirmed COVID-19-infected patients. Two midwives had contracted long COVID-19 (COVID-19 symptoms persisting for months), with one having to take a long-term leave and the other shifting to part-time work. Neither had been able to access WorkSafeBC support, and both were greatly concerned about their financial stability.

BEING ESSENTIAL

For midwives, the pandemic highlighted a lack of awareness and recognition of their contributions to the broader health system. Midwives' higher risk of infection was rarely recognized because they were grouped with other professions within the allied healthcare category, such as dieticians, who could shift to exclusively virtual care. Numerous participants pointed out that the minister of health did not include midwives when he thanked frontline workers in media statements. One midwife described the hurt this omission caused, "[L]ike just mention us. Just acknowledge us. I think it's huge. Like that would go so far even now." Others expressed feeling "forgotten as first-line providers," with their efforts largely unrecognized, unsupported, and

undervalued by health leadership. As a result, celebrations of other
essential workers were seen as almost insulting. Midwives described
receiving health authority emails about the supports provided to
officially recognized essential healthcare workers, such as pandemic
pay top-ups, which they did not qualify for, as "traumatic" and
"demoralizing." A participant noted that such emails reinforced the
perception that "nobody even thinks about like how harmful that
would be to receive an email that discriminates against your compensation." Midwives frequently commented on the contrast between
their experiences and the heroic images prevalent during the initial
months of the pandemic:

> We're getting these emails that are talking about "Physician
> and nurse compensation for your heroic efforts." ... Meanwhile,
> everyone's struggling. All the clinic owners are struggling.
> There's so much burnout ... Most of us recognize we're frontline
> healthcare workers in a pandemic, but [there is] this complete
> invisibility of the work that we do.

Because midwives are designated as allied healthcare workers, they
did not initially receive PPE through BC government supply chains.
Instead, they had to source PPE themselves, which was difficult during
the first few months of the pandemic because of shortages: "We have
no PPE. We're actually begging our clients to supply us. We have no
quarantine pay, no hazard pay. We are really struggling here. And we
really want to keep offering our care because we're keeping healthy
people out of the hospital." Midwives described sewing their own
masks, washing and reusing gloves, and asking clients to bring their
own PPE. They ordered from Amazon, used hospital connections to
secretly access PPE, sought out sanitizer from local distilleries, and
received glove donations from tattoo parlours. Not only did having
to patch together PPE supplies take up a lot of time, but when they
couldn't find what they needed, they were unable to protect themselves
or the families they served. One midwife explained, "You need to
understand that we birth. We get covered in fluid. We get spat on.
We get vomited on. We have amniotic fluid on us, poop, everything. We
are out in the community. You maybe don't know we're here, but this
is what we're doing. We need PPE." Due to the lack of PPE supplies,
midwives were highly concerned about contracting COVID-19 and
transmitting it to clients and family members. One midwife, who

worked specifically with populations made vulnerable, had provided care to four COVID-19-positive parents in the past eight months, from one of whom she had contracted COVID-19.

Midwives noted that many of their fellow healthcare workers were also frustrated by midwives' lack of access to PPE. They recounted birth centre managers, patient coordinators, and obstetricians sourcing PPE for them and advocating for including them in PPE planning. In one community, midwives had written to their MLA (member of the provincial legislative assembly) about their lack of access to PPE, and the MLA had sourced PPE for them. After the first few months of the pandemic and in response to midwives' advocacy and support from these allies, most hospitals began providing PPE to midwives for home births. However, midwives continued to have to source their own supplies for regular checkups with pregnant people and for home visits to check in on newborns. Plus, midwives could only access PPE for home births from the hospital, with some having to get permission for each PPE request, a system that did not take the unpredictable and urgent nature of labour into account. One midwife commented that such policies "reflected a lack of understanding of what we do and who we are." Another said the need to request PPE was demoralizing: "this constant feeling of like having to remind people that we're there and that we work there." Midwives also did not have access to the financial assistance provided to doctors to improve the safety of their offices or purchase equipment to provide virtual care. They spoke of wanting to install better air filtration systems in their clinics but not being able to afford them. They were also ineligible for the pandemic pay provided to essential workers such as nurses and LTC care aides. This added insult to the injury of already feeling underpaid and unrecognized.

The experience of one midwife illustrates the contradiction between not being considered essential, and therefore not provided with resources, while providing essential health care. This midwife worked in a practice that provided services to urban and Indigenous parents, as well as those with complex medical histories and housing challenges. Within the first year of the pandemic, the practice had four clients and two babies test positive for COVID-19. The midwife also contracted COVID-19 from a client. She explained:

I was in isolation in quarantine for two weeks over Christmas in a hotel on my holidays and it was very unpleasant. And the

additional stress of – like the financial stress of being in a
hotel, because that was the only way I could isolate effectively
in my home, having to inform my roommates, having to
inform my partner. I was calling WorkSafe, and I was calling
the Midwi[ves] Association of BC to ask about benefits and
like what's going to happen if I'm really sick. Like do I have – like
I pay into sick benefits. I pay into WorkSafe. This is like a worksite exposure. Am I going to have any kind of coverage if this
is a long-term issue? And they both said I have no coverage,
no protection, despite paying into these benefits, and of course,
I was pretty scared, just because it's kind of unpredictable.

In the midst of sorting out her own care and isolation arrangements,
the midwife got a call from the public health agency.

Like six hours after I got off the phone with public health,
they called me back and they asked me to go and do a home
visit for the person that I'd contracted COVID from – and I was
like, 'I'm in quarantine. I actually can't do that." And also, this
is so problematic that you think that this is appropriate that
you're calling me, like you just told me to quarantine. I'm in
the first twenty-four hours of being sick. I don't have sick
benefits. I'm supposed to be travelling to go and see this person
and also, like you're capitalizing on the relationship that I have
with this high-risk youth. You know like, the fact that I do
deeply care about this person and the relationship that we have
and the fact that I know she's sick. It just felt so manipulative
as well, because … they're like, 'Well, nobody else is going to
see her, because she has COVID. If you don't see her, we don't
know when the next time she's going to be seen is." And I was
like 'I'm so sick. Like I have a fever.'

Midwives lived the contradiction of doing frontline, high-risk work
without recognition or the most basic level of support. One reflected,
"It just feels like everyone is kind of telling us, like, keep providing
your service. In fact, provide more of your service, but without any
help, any compensation, and we'll just keep treating you like shit."
They described the experience of being praised for their frontline work
without being properly integrated into the health system and protected
as "gaslighting" and being "hung out to dry."

MENTAL WELLNESS, MORAL DISTRESS, AND BURNOUT

Midwives experienced moral distress related to their perceived inability to provide quality care in the context of the pandemic. They worried that protocols limiting in-person visits would negatively affect the quality of care because they were unable to see clients and newborns regularly. In one tragic incident, a midwife had belatedly identified the termination of a fetus's heartbeat because she had had to hold virtual visits – an outcome she held herself personally responsible for although she had been following public health advice. Midwives further described high levels of uncertainty and distress during the initial months of the pandemic when little research was available on the effects of COVID-19 on pregnancy and birth. Despite their efforts to stay up to date on emerging research and new policies, they often felt helpless when faced with questions from expectant and new parents they could not answer. Constantly changing protocols and hospital rules meant they did not always know how best to prepare pregnant people, and they shared clients' frustrations with the unknown and the uncertainty.

The strict protocols required to contain COVID-19 often felt contradictory to the relationship-based, whole-of-person approach inherent in midwifery care. As the editor of a midwifery journal wrote, "For many midwives, visualizing the care we provide during labor and birth likely conjures images of a caring professional face-to-face with a patient, holding a hand, rubbing a back, fostering the initial bonds of a new family" (Murphy 2020, 299). Midwives explained how having to rush through appointments, maintain distance from clients, and remind others of COVID-19 protocols made them feel, "[T]his isn't midwifery care." In particular, they struggled with regulations against physical contact. One noted, "[I]t's also been hard because I know that I'm not giving the type of care that I would really love to give sometimes. Because it's not words that people need, it's touch a lot of the time and we can't touch anymore, we can't hug anymore." Another commented on feeling guilty for the emotional distance created during a delivery due to faces having to be covered, and how she tried to express "love and encouragement" with her eyes. In some situations, the moral obligation to provide quality care ultimately led midwives to break COVID-19 regulations and compromise their own health and safety. For example,

In labour, rubbing somebody's back or just feeling her arm and smoothing her hair out of her face, that's what I do. Those little things make the care "care," not just a person standing in a room. And so, when you're asked to just be this distant person in the room ... I think midwives pretty much fail at that. We just can't really do that. And so, that's just the risk, right? You take that risk.

Taking such risks led to some midwives feeling moral distress about potentially contracting or spreading COVID-19. This distress was heightened by the lack of access to adequate PPE during the initial months of the pandemic. One midwife described an instance of having two home births in one night but only enough PPE for one and so having to decide whether to reuse the PPE or ask the second person in labour to go to the hospital. She opted for the latter and felt guilty that she was not able to ensure the type of birth the family preferred.

Impediments to practising relationship-based care affected midwives' job satisfaction, because the "joyful moments" of chatting with parents and playing with children and other "things that fill the cup" were prohibited. Without such positive returns on their work, midwives felt increasingly burned out. One midwife reflected, "People's experience of midwifery care has really changed. That is a place where we find high work satisfaction – is connection with clients and it's one of the key factors that motivates people ... [There is] not the same level of job satisfaction in terms of relationship with our clients and now they have burnt-out healthcare providers." This reduction in job satisfaction made the challenges of the pandemic harder to bear.

When midwives felt physically or mentally ill, they faced a moral conflict over taking time off (in addition to the financial barriers as discussed above) as was recommended, recognizing the increased strain it would put on colleagues given that they worked in small teams whose patient caseloads were usually already at capacity. One midwife stated, "If you're sick, you're putting some heavy weight on your teammates." Another noted, "[W]e have to just make this choice [on whether to leave work] when we have symptoms because it's the right thing to do, but it's hugely damaging from a like a team perspective, a burnout perspective." One midwife described her practice trying to come up with continuity plans when a team member became sick, but "it got so complex, so quickly that we couldn't do it." Feeling it wasn't possible to leave work even though she was struggling with poor mental health, another midwife described constantly measuring her mental wellness using a burnout scorecard she had received from a nurse, just to make sure she wouldn't be a danger to others, instead of taking time off.

Midwives' ability to self-care was inhibited by their lack of extended health benefits. One midwife spoke of going into debt so she could access counselling:

> Like I also have increased my counselling in the last few months cause I'm like, "you know what, we can't afford it, but I also can't afford not to do it," so we're just going to go into debt and I'm putting it all on my credit card because I need to speak to someone because it's just too much.

While midwives came up with such strategies to cope with the stressors of providing care during a pandemic, they recognized that most strategies were unsustainable, with one midwife noting, "I just feel like I couldn't handle the level of work," and another stating, "[J]ust when you think it just can't get any more intense ... there's another wave." They described burnout as the culmination of a lack of recognition and support for their profession, accompanied by reduced emotional fulfillment from their careers, in a context of increased risk:

> We lost two very experienced incredible midwives in the last year and a half ... It's almost like when you're in a midlife crisis, midwives are going through that. They're trying to figure out how to make this sustainable or to find a Plan B. There's this crossroad right now. I'm hearing everyone talk about a Plan B, myself included.

Identifying the signs of burnout had a multiplier effect in that many midwives then felt guilty for considering leaving the profession, feeling a responsibility to both their colleagues and pregnant people seeking midwifery care. Participants spoke of how the need to "just keep going on" was ingrained in the midwifery profession but was also unsustainable: "[I]f we don't put ourselves first and take care of ourselves and make sure there's sustainability in the profession, we're not helping our clients long-term." Others described a "martyr complex" where midwives continued to work despite the harm to their well-being and the lack of support because "we don't do it for the benefits, or we don't do it for the pay." Reflecting such thinking, another noted, "we will keep working in the pandemic, and we'll keep working as underpaid people, we'll keep being undervalued by our communities, our hospital, and we'll keep doing it because we love what we do." This commitment, while admirable, also had midwives working to the breaking point – with some repeatedly taking burnout surveys and going into debt to access mental health care.

POWER

Many midwives felt that their peripheral position within the healthcare system reflected the feminization of their profession, being largely characterized by women midwives caring for women clients. In many ways, midwifery was doubly feminized because it was conducted by women for feminized people, and this led to the healthcare system neglecting them. One midwife explained, "[T]here's actually been very little planning and thought [about integrating midwifery into pandemic response], and it's because it's women. It's because it's women and it's because it's kids." Another noted, "[I]t just really feels like we're so undervalued and the fact that it's a profession that is dominated by women and ... we care for women or like child-bearing people." Another positioned midwifery within broader social norms around gender roles: "[T]here is a clear association with how women are treated in our society, because of the fact that this alternately affects women and that we're a female-dominated profession, it's a female healthcare issue." In a doubly feminized profession, midwives often felt doubly marginalized.

For example, because midwives weren't integrated into the healthcare system, decisions on reproductive care during the pandemic were made without their input. Almost all participants cited the same two examples of this exclusion during the initial months of the COVID-19 response: restrictions on home births and midwives' participation in Caesarean sections. About 30 per cent of midwife-attended births occur in the home, and home births attended by midwives have been found to be as safe as hospital births (Nethery et al. 2021). The initial ban on home births reflected fears about whether COVID-19 protocols could be maintained in the home. However, at the same time, more parents were requesting home births to avoid hospitals, which were seen as riskier sites for COVID-19, and midwives quickly adapted COVID-19 protocols to home births, arguing that they could be just as safe, if not safer. Non-hospital births rose from 1.74 per cent in 2019 to 2.12 per cent of births in 2020, across Canada, largely due to parents' desire to avoid hospitals during the pandemic (Statistics Canada 2021). The guidance against home births contradicted the increase in demand for home births that midwives were experiencing and their commitment to pregnant peoples' autonomy. One midwife explained:

> Leadership basically advised that we stop doing home births. That was a big stretch for us because we were getting more people asking for home births ... We had to do some shuffling and changing to become more involved in the discussion. And to let them know that because of our philosophy of informed choice discussions, it's not really our choice to stop doing home births ... It felt like a huge paradigm shift for them to understand the way we worked a little bit more and for us to get a seat at the table.

Within two months, midwives successfully convinced the health authorities of the safety of home births, enabling parents to choose the type of birth they felt most comfortable with.

In some hospitals, midwives were also initially excluded from Caesarean procedures. During Caesarean sections, midwives provide advice and comfort to parents, support physical checks of the infant, and ensure that the infant and parent bond as soon as safely possible. During what can be a traumatic surgery, midwives provide continuity of care and emotional support. Those were initially seen as unnecessary because hospitals aimed to reduce the number of people in a room and therefore the risk of COVID-19 transmission. Midwives felt this prioritization devalued their contributions: "Initially, they weren't letting us into the operating room as midwives ... Just another way that they kind of told us that the work we do is undervalued. That there really wasn't a role for us in the OR, which just goes to show, I think, on a more systematic level, how much people don't care about women's emotional health and the experience that birth is." Midwives committed a substantial amount of time to advocate for a change in this policy, successfully convincing most hospitals within a few months to allow them to be present during Caesareans.

Midwives described widely varying participation within hospital decision-making around pandemic protocols, reflecting midwifery's lack of formalized integration into hospital-based reproductive care. Many reported that it was hard to get "a seat at the table," noting that they had to "work for it" and "do some shuffling." Others felt that "even when we sat at tables and tried to be part of committees, we never felt like our voices were heard. We didn't feel like there was much difference whether we were there or not." They described "having to go above and beyond" to have their concerns heard and often feeling they were "an afterthought." Midwives felt that there was a widespread lack of understanding of the role of midwifery within the hospital system. One midwife had to spend a lot of time in COVID-19 planning meetings trying to explain what midwives do, which contributed to her emotional exhaustion: "They think that we're just cuddling babies all day. There's just so much behind-the-scenes stuff that we're doing all the time, right?" This lack of awareness meant midwives' expertise was not always acknowledged, even when it could have strengthened the health system's pandemic response. One midwife reflected, "[I]t would be nice if we were first of all recognized that we actually have a lot of skills and things to contribute."

A smaller number noted that hospital decision-makers sought out their insights and requested that they participate in decision-making bodies. One midwife reported that the family practice division in her hospital intentionally included midwives in meetings and that, based on this example, doctors had also started asking midwives for input into decision-making. Some midwives played leadership roles in developing COVID-19 policies, such as in planning around Caesarean section procedures. Others were part of teams developing precautions for COVID-19-positive parents. While enabling midwives to have a voice, such involvement added to their workload; unlike the hospital staff and physicians, midwives were not paid for the time they spent on such committees. One midwife reflected on the time she dedicated to COVID-19-related decision-making processes at the hospital: "[I]t's great to get involved, and it is helpful to know what things are in different levels, but that was crazy. Like I can handle a lot, and that felt excessive." Several noted that they could not participate in such forums because they were already being overwhelmed with increased work burdens and unpaid care responsibilities.

Midwives' marginalization within decision-making structures was viewed not so much as purposeful but as a result of not being hospital employees and few in number, and due to other healthcare providers' lack of understanding of their role. One midwife noted, "I feel marginalized as a midwife and as a midwife leader ... COVID-19 has amplified that. It shows that there's no system for midwives because it's created for physicians and nurses. We're just too small. And they're not going to start new systems for us, and they won't let us join existing systems." However, the pressures of the pandemic were viewed as adding "fuel to the fire," compelling midwives to become involved in advocacy efforts when new protocols compromised midwifery values around informed choice. Some midwives were hopeful that their advocacy efforts, paired with increased awareness of their valuable work, would lead to stronger support and decision-making opportunities in the future.

CONCLUSION

Throughout history, midwifery has been a site of revolutionary struggle for women's rights and autonomy for pregnant people. Within the crisis of the pandemic, midwives continued to advocate for themselves and for those to whom they provide care. As demand for midwifery care peaked, midwives fought for access to PPE, the right to be present during Caesareans, and to offer home births. For their efforts, often expended at great cost to themselves and their families, they received little acknowledgement and no pandemic pay or similar supports. Like other healthcare workers, they faced heightened sources of stress and moral distress. Yet, unlike other healthcare workers, they did not have access to mental health support or paid sick days. The feminization of midwifery meant that it continued to be positioned on the periphery of the health system. Having to wage battle against both a virus and their marginalization within the health system added greatly to midwives' workloads, further increasing their risk of burnout.

To counter these trends, midwives first asked to be recognized as essential healthcare workers and to receive the same support as other frontline healthcare professionals, such as pandemic pay, funds to adapt clinics during emergencies, and sick benefits. In the case of future infectious disease outbreaks, they noted that midwives need direct access to BC government PPE supply chains, given how high risk their work is. The shortage of midwives and the risk of attrition in the industry require further interventions to support midwives' mental health and work-life balance. Standardized approaches to including midwifery representation in leadership and decision-making can help overcome the lack of awareness about their role in the health system. Without such reforms, there is a real risk of a decline in midwifery services, which would greatly reduce the options for quality care for pregnant people and children in the province.

7

Nobody Is Clapping for Us

Early Childhood Educators

You know, there were a lot of like, you know, they're clapping for
the nurses, they're clapping for all the essential workers, but they never
mention us. Like, we're taking care of your children and yet nobody's
clapping for us ... And I felt like, hey, hello, you can thank us too,
we don't mind if you want to thank us.

Early childhood educator

INTRODUCTION

In early March 2020, my daughter and I entered her daycare facility
and saw one of the educators trying to take the temperature of a child
who was sitting on her lap. Two other kids hung off her back, and a
couple more crowded around. She was asking them to back up, but
as they were only three or four years old, their curiosity overwhelmed
their listening ability. I paused and asked, "Should I be worried?"
There were no COVID-19 protocols in place at this point, though case
numbers in BC were rising. The educator looked up, glancing at
the thermometer with an expression that suggested she didn't have the
energy to deal with both the excitable kids and an anxious parent.
"No, no it's fine. He doesn't have a fever," she said as she gave the
worried-looking preschooler a squeeze and sent him off to play.
I hugged my daughter goodbye but left feeling anxious about her safety
and, at first, frustrated with the chaos I'd witnessed. "They clearly
don't know what to do," I vented to a colleague. Then I remembered

that educators are not public health professionals trained in pandemic management and that the educator sitting with a feverish child on her lap, surrounded by other children, was probably the person most at risk. It wasn't her fault there was no pandemic plan in place for child-care centres. A week later, I withdrew my daughter from child care, and a week after that, childcare centres across the province closed to all but the children of essential workers.

That same week, while my parents watched my daughter, I began planning the Gender and COVID-19 Project, considering which groups of women I would seek out for interviews. The image of that educator, trying to take one kid's temperature while surrounded by other kids and being questioned by an anxious parent, came to mind. I knew the profession was female-dominated (over 95 per cent of educators are women), including a disproportionate number of racialized and newcomer women (Uppal and Savage 2021). The partial closure of childcare centres had suddenly made parents, employers, and the government aware of their importance, but their location, at the time outside of education and health systems, meant they rarely featured in discussions of essential work. Curious, I reached out through contacts with the Coalition of Child Care Advocates of BC, which advocates for accessible and affordable child care in the province, and which I had been involved with as a volunteer a few years earlier. Through that network and social media posts, I got in touch with nine educators and interviewed them in May and June 2020. All were working in licensed facilities, some in smaller private centres and others in large non-profit-run organizations.

Though this is one of the smaller data sets included in this book, I am grateful I get to share these women's experiences because, as they themselves point out, they have largely been ignored. At the time of writing, the experiences of educators during the pandemic have hardly been researched or covered by the media. Most commentaries and reports on COVID-19 childcare challenges focus on the experiences of working mothers, ignoring the experiences of those who provide care so that we can work (Wallace and Goodyear-Grant 2020). These seemingly progressive discussions about the effects on mothers' careers can reinforce notions of care work as mothers' work (as opposed to fathers') while rendering the work of paid care providers invisible (Powell et al. 2020). This happens despite the majority of children in Canada receiving a combination of paid and unpaid care (Halfon and Langford 2015). Furthermore, as is evident in the other chapters of this book, many essential workers are parents who need child care to do their jobs – therefore, all other essential labour relies on child care. It is the home base from which all other frontline work is launched.

As discussed in chapter 5, BC's childcare sector is "chaotic and unorganized" because of a historical lack of investment, a mix of provider types (including for-profit and not-for-profit, institutional and home-based, licensed and unlicensed), varying working conditions for educators, and a lack of accessibility for parents (Milne 2016). Early childhood education in Canada is characterized by low pay, no benefits, and little recognition of its contributions to society. It is viewed more as a service than a profession, despite a growing number of educators earning post-secondary qualifications (Halfon and Langford 2015). This context started to change in 2018, when the newly elected BC New Democratic Party (NDP) increased investments in child care with promises to fund more spaces and reduce fees. Despite these initial steps, when COVID-19 emerged in early 2020 the sector was still very much characterized by fragmentation, high costs, and inaccessibility, with many childcare educators making less than a living wage ($20 an hour in 2020 in the Lower Mainland of BC, where the research was conducted) (Macdonald and Friendly 2021). Unique among Canadian provinces, the BC government did not order childcare centres closed when it announced a public health emergency in March 2020 and closed schools and other services. While a few centres closed temporarily on their own initiative, most followed government directives, asking families who could do so to keep their children at home, but remaining open for the children of essential workers. As a result, educators had to quickly adapt to providing child care in the midst of a public health crisis.

THE QUADRUPLE BURDEN

When the province closed schools due to COVID-19 on 17 March 2020, the Early Childhood Educators of BC (ECEBC) requested that childcare facilities also be closed until clear health guidelines were in place. An educator explained, "[T]he ECEBC wanted government to close daycares because there were no standards in place." However, this request was denied on the basis of arguments that child care was required for essential workers, so educators instead asked for information on how to ensure health and safety in childcare settings. One explained,

A couple of us had a phone call with the public health authority about this and said, you know, it would be really good if you as a medical authority would say, here's what the research shows about how children figure in this whole thing. People were saying, like, children are going to be super-spreaders and all this kind of stuff, which didn't seem to be true ... So we kept trying to pull those things together and saying, you know, this is an emergency. How does child care fit into it?

However, educators felt that "there wasn't a lot of direct communication as far as, okay, you can have these many children in your centre, you can have this many staff. There wasn't a lot of directives, it was just very vague, and you were sort of left hanging." Without clear information, educators had to develop their own protocols, spending time researching and trying to make sense of the latest medical information while caring for young children. An educator explained, "[W]e changed everything," including no longer letting parents in, taking children's temperatures, and removing toys that were hard to clean.

The information provided was often conflicting, with different guidance from the Ministry of Education, Ministry of Health, health authorities, and child care licensing officers. An educator explained that she got two different sets of advice when a child arrived at her centre with a fever. Educators reported having to come up with their own policies for wearing masks, using gloves, and cleaning. In one case, an educator realized she had been potentially exposed to COVID-19 because her daughter, who lived with her, worked in a care home that was experiencing an outbreak. When she told her colleagues, they were not sure if she could come to work or if they should close the centre. One manager noted that while she received emails from the Ministry of Children and Family Development about best practices for preventing the spread of COVID-19, she did not get responses to inquiries about where to get PPE and cleaning supplies. She further noted that one of the best practices suggested was for educators who were sick to take ten days off or get a COVID-19 test, unrealistic in an industry that was understaffed and where people got sick all the time. One centre manager reflected, "This is why we wanted the daycare shut until we could sit down ... We are ready to help figure out these protocols, figure out these standards that need to be met because we know what we're doing."

Educators described feeling exhausted by the need to keep up an "upbeat and happy front" for the children while struggling with uncertainty. The emotional labour of maintaining a positive and comforting environment for children was substantial, and educators described returning home overwhelmed at the end of the day:

> I think there is a lot of hidden anxiety, you know, we're all, yeah, I'm fine, I'm fine, I'm fine. And then, all of a sudden, you'll be doing something else, and you'll burst into tears for no reason. You're like, okay, why did I cry … It's, like, you know, you're going through trauma, you go into survival mode. And at this point, I don't think any of us really understand what this is doing to us emotionally and physically, until we're past it and we can look back on it. I think a lot of us are going through trauma without even, at this point, really recognizing it.

Other than increased cleaning and ensuring physical distancing from parents, few prevention measures were available to educators who were, at this point in the pandemic, being advised against wearing masks because of concerns it would scare children and impede communication. As a result, as one educator put it, "we are people working without any protection really. We try, and we have our protocols for when the parents drop off, but sometimes, you know, you come within that six feet when you're taking that child from the other parent." Another noted, "[O]ur families are lovely people, but I don't think they realize. Sometimes they just walk in or drop off a kid with a cold." While educators invested substantial time and labour in keeping up to date on COVID-19 information and developing COVID-19 precautions, they struggled to maintain health and safety protocols.

Over half of the educators interviewed were newcomers to Canada, reflecting the broader field within which immigrants and non-permanent residents are overrepresented. In 2021, 28 per cent of childcare workers were immigrants or non-permanent residents, compared with 23 per cent of all other workers (Uppal and Savage 2021). Newcomer educators faced particular challenges during COVID-19. For example, newcomers reported being more concerned than the general population about their health and maintaining social ties during the initial months of the pandemic (Larochelle-Côté and Uppal 2020). Many did not have the same family and social support networks as those who had been in Canada longer, which limited their coping strategies. For example, when a newcomer educator had to isolate due to a potential exposure, she had no one to bring her groceries or other necessities and thus had to rely on expensive food delivery services, which increased the costs of her isolation.

For newcomers responsible for the care of others, the occupational risk combined with the lack of established social support networks multiplied the potential negative effects of COVID-19 infection. An educator who was also a newcomer single mom decided to leave her job because the risk of getting sick and being unable to care for her son outweighed the economic risk of lost employment:

I was scared I was going to get sick from the air because at that time like they say it's very powerful, it's going to kill you and I was afraid. They closed the school, and I can take [my son] to daycare with me, but if I take him to the daycare he's going to be in contact with more adults, more grown-ups and he's going to get sick. I was so afraid. At that moment I felt safe at home because I know I'm going to be in control of what he touch, what he eats. Because my fear is that like if I get sick, who is going to look after my son, because I don't have no one. I don't have family or relatives.

Now subsisting on employment insurance, this mother spent most of her income on rent, to the point that she had to rely on food baskets from a charity. She was further aware that giving up her educator position would now affect her long-term opportunities, disrupting the Canadian work experience she was trying to build. At the time of the interview, she worried that when schools reopened, she would no longer have access to after-school care for her son. The childcare centre she had worked at had provided it, and without after-school care she was not sure if she could find another job.

Many educators also had elder-care responsibilities, which became complicated because of the combination of their occupational risk and seniors' increased risk of severe health outcomes from infection. One educator spoke of the challenges of caring for her elderly mother with dementia. The mother was on a waitlist for a full-service long-term-care residence, but the process had been stalled by heightened concerns about COVID-19 outbreaks in long-term-care facilities. The educator described driving over an hour just to see her mother through the window, unable to go in because she feared potentially transmitting COVID-19. She would leave groceries on the doorstep and call her mother on the phone, but often her mother did not recognize her. She explained, "She used to recognize me when I was there with her. Now I'm terrified she never will again. That when this is finally over, she will never recognize me again." The educator talked about her mother, during a phone call a few nights earlier, describing abominable pain she was having, which the educator identified as the symptoms of a urinary tract infection. The educator called an ambulance for her mother but was unable to accompany her to the hospital because of COVID-19 restrictions. She reflected, "[T]he doctor said I saved her life by calling 911, but I don't know. I can only do so little."

For both these women, the risk of working without protection was incompatible with providing care for their dependents. One resolved this conflict by leaving her paid care work, the other by restricting her unpaid care abilities. Both incurred costs for these forced decisions – one lost employment and income, the other paid with increased anxiety and grief.

BEING ESSENTIAL

Educators were genuinely surprised to be recognized as essential workers. Because the sector had previously been neglected, one educator "thought it might be a mistake. That they would take it back and say, 'oops, no, we didn't mean it.'" She noted, on the one hand, "this is a huge thing for the childcare community. To be called essential workers." The centrality of child care to families and the economy was finally beginning to be realized, which, as another educator explained, "was not new to any of us, but it was new to certain people. Like bankers. You know, people that said, holy shit, you know, childcare is really important. The economy depends on child care. Like, duh." Others noted a new recognition from parents that "we are not just babysitters."

On the other hand, a disconnect between the title of essential and the continued lack of support heightened educators' pre-COVID-19 frustrations: "I feel like, especially in the beginning, there were so many educators that were angry that they were considered essential workers and not a lot of resources were given to them, or information was not given to them." While formally listed as essential, most educators still felt that their contribution to the response was devalued. For example, almost all specifically mentioned the evening neighbourhood clapping and noisemaking, which was done as a way to thank healthcare workers during lockdown: "You know, there were a lot of like, you know, they're clapping for the nurses, they're clapping for all the essential workers, but they never mention us. Like, we're taking care of your children and yet nobody's clapping for us ... And I felt like, hey, hello, you can thank us too, we don't mind if you want to thank us." Despite the increased recognition of the centrality of child care, educators felt that the lack of acknowledgment and appreciation reflected pre-pandemic attitudes toward child care as a service rather than a profession: "I feel like we're still sort of being taken for granted a bit," and "I still find a little bit that we're not valued as much as maybe we should be sometimes. And I mean, I've felt that for thirty years, I've never from the public felt very much valued."

Educators further felt that the risk they assumed went unacknowledged. One woman stated, "I don't think that people are really recognizing how much we're putting ourselves at risk." Another noted, "I think in the beginning there were kind of just the response I heard – and I felt a little bit too, like, okay, you're educators, can you just go back and take care of these children. I think the fear that a lot of people had going back, wasn't addressed. They just felt like they weren't being heard, and I think that just gave them some – they just felt sort of marginalized and just kind of not valued." Educators frequently compared their level of risk to that of other essential workers, whose children they were taking care of: "We're not even allowed to wear masks, because it could scare the children. Even hospital workers, they're still having protection, but for us in the field, we're very, very exposed, because we can't wear gloves, we can't wear masks." They frequently contrasted their experiences with those of teachers: "Like you have a desk to sit at. OK, you can isolate. Well, there's no desks in child care." Many recognized a contradiction between the responses in the school and childcare sectors:

It was interesting, though, to see that disconnect between the school system and child care, because, you know, there's all this thing about masks, and how to protect the teachers and physical distancing in a kindergarten room ... But then in the childcare facility across the street, there are four-year-olds that are, you know, in a totally different situation.

These differences reinforced educators' impression that as essential workers they were second-class:

> I think that was one of the things where a lot of the – back
> in the spring, the people in the childcare sector, you know,
> the ECEs, the workers, were saying, well, what are we? Like
> chopped liver? You know, like, the teachers are important,
> we're not important? You know? They closed school[s] before
> child care practically everywhere in Canada because school
> is school and child care [is] well … well, what is that? Like,
> you know. It's this recognition kind of thing. Besides making,
> you know, low wages and, you know, all of that kind of stuff,
> we aren't worth protecting.

The Coalition of Child Care Advocates of BC and allies had long lobbied for child care to be included under the Ministry of Education to promote public oversight of the sector and improve working conditions, a request that was reiterated in the context of the pandemic (and eventually achieved in 2022). However, at the time of the interviews, the labelling of educators as essential highlighted their lack of support and recognition compared with the education and health sectors.

MENTAL HEALTH, MORAL DISTRESS, AND BURNOUT

All the educators interviewed spoke of how a lack of clear guidelines and concerns about the risk of infection caused them high levels of stress and anxiety. A centre manager explained, "Like staff really didn't know if they were going to get it and die, for example, if they went to work." While concerned about their own safety, educators were particularly anxious about how to keep the children in their care safe. One educator explained: "My anxiety skyrocket[ed]. I couldn't sleep … I had two small children and we were in the play area. One was licking the ground and one was licking the railing. I couldn't keep that sanitized." Educators described their anxiety over decisions about what toys to allow based on whether they could be sanitized and the constant self-monitoring of personal hygiene and physical distance they had to practise.

Educators experienced moral dilemmas related to balancing COVID-19 precautions with the need to provide care, often through physical contact, to young children: "[W]e are huggers. I want to hug children ... Now I'm always pulling back, and it hurts." Educators spoke of how physical distancing requirements created conflicting feelings of guilt; for example, if a child fell and hurt themselves, they felt guilty whether they picked up the child or did not. They further described physical distancing requirements affecting their ability to support one another: "We're physical people, ECEs. I try to keep a distance from my colleagues but it's hard. One was upset so I put my arm around her and then I realized I shouldn't but ... it's the way we are." The tension between their role as care providers, which necessitated physical contact, and physical distancing requirements resulted in educators constantly questioning themselves and feeling guilty for providing either too much or too little care.

Educators faced moral uncertainty about their desire to keep childcare spaces as safe as possible given the limited and constantly changing information available at the time while also maintaining normalcy and a sense of calm for the children in their care. One described trying to teach children to maintain physical distance: "It's very hard. If children see other friends – they want to go to other children, right? And they want to stay together. So, we tried to separate them. Like during the lunchtime and then snack time, and then naptime, but it's hard." The inherent conflict between the safety recommendations and the requirements of providing care to small children meant educators felt that they and the children were at high risk of contracting COVID-19, leading to further anxiety. That anxiety affected educators' ability to sleep, their stress levels, and their emotional well-being.

POWER

During the initial months of the pandemic, ECEBC held town halls and workshops with educators to answer questions and hear concerns, which ECEBC relayed to the BC government. A participant in these meetings recounted how educators' knowledge of the sector could have been combined with public health expertise to enhance child and educator safety: "They said [to government], ask us. We are here to be asked." However, respondents had the impression that they were not listened to. Not only did the province keep centres open despite educators' requests for temporary closure, but educators' questions about PPE and protocols often went unanswered, as did offers to provide educator expertise in developing provincial COVID-19 protocols for childcare settings.

As a result, the burden of developing COVID-19 policies fell on individual centres and educators, a burden that was not borne equally in a sector described pre-pandemic as fragmented, chaotic, unstable, and disorganized (Macdonald and Friendly 2021; Milne 2016). Large centres run by non-profit organizations had boards that were able to share decision-making responsibilities, whereas in smaller facilities decisions fell on one or two people. One educator from a large community-based facility described those working in small private centres contacting her for advice:

> I have a lot more people involved, and I have a bigger covering. You know, so [Organization] came in and they had their policies and they made me feel confident. I had [Organization], but they [smaller centre staff] didn't, they only could rely on the communication from the government, so they were calling me and just going, like, what do we do? Like, do we have these families, are they allowed to come in the centre? They felt that there were a lot of unanswered questions.

An educator from a small private centre reiterated this concern: "So even between the group daycares and family daycares that distinction, like I felt like some of the things that were coming out were more targeted to the group daycares versus family daycare, versus – like it should just be all daycares, right? For anyone who's taking care of kids you know." The fragmentation of the sector inhibited the government's ability to communicate effectively with educators and therefore compromised children's safety.

Because of a lack of safety guidelines, some educators considered not returning to work. One centre manager noted that three of her staff of six quit because they didn't feel safe. However, most did not have that option. In 2019, the average hourly wage for educators was $20 per hour, just equal to the living wage of $20 in the Lower Mainland of BC. As noted above, one educator who did leave work, fearing infection, later had to rely on food baskets from a charity. Others explained that they considered leaving work, but that the financial risk outweighed the health risk. One educator whose age put her at risk for more severe COVID-19-related outcomes explained: "So for me, it came down to a financial decision. Because I couldn't be laid off and collect any EI [employment insurance] or anything else, I chose to come to work." Another noted that because both her adult children had lost work and were now living with her, she could not manage on employment insurance or CERB. There was also ambiguity about whether those who left work due to fear of COVID-19 would be eligible for CERB, since guidelines stated that it was only available to those who had lost work, not those who had "chosen" not to work out of fear of exposure. Another educator explained,

> In the beginning my husband was, like, you're not going back, you're staying, home, this is ridiculous. You shouldn't be going back. And I was, like, oh, you know, should I go back, shouldn't I go back? Like, kind of on the fence about it. But, so for myself, you know, I talked to my employers, and I was, like, okay, what if I don't choose to come back, what are my options? And it wasn't an option to be laid off. If we chose not to take the work offered, that would mean just being at home and not collecting any money.

Having to take time off because of illness or to isolate further contributed to educators' financial insecurity. An educator who developed symptoms was told to get tested and isolate until she received the results. She had to wait ten days for test results, using up all her paid sick days for the year, noting that she was "fortunate" because her wait time extended into the planned spring break closure, "otherwise I wouldn't have been paid for the second week." Considering that 40 per cent of educators in the province do not have paid sick days, many would have lost income in such a situation (Milne 2016).

Lacking a voice in decision-making and lacking a choice about employment conditions combined to force educators to remain on the front lines of the response without any corresponding support or guidance. In response, educators gathered virtually to share good practices and develop common messages. One respondent noted that the energy within the discussions was so filled with anger that she felt that "there is going to be some sort of uprising" due to the frustrations educators were dealing with. Another noted, "I do think that the pandemic has given us an opportunity to kind of transform child care. And I've noticed this coming from the field, you know, the sector, more than I would have ever thought." Indeed, educators and their allies have used the pandemic to highlight their essential role, with both the federal and provincial governments since announcing major investments in the sector.

CONCLUSION

While designated as essential workers and assuming a high degree of risk because of a lack of safety precautions and guidance, educators had little say in decision-making at the provincial level during the initial months of the pandemic. Their request to temporarily close facilities was ignored, because their labour was deemed critical to provide care to the children of other essential workers. While denied a voice at the provincial level, they were expected to take on the responsibility of ensuring safety within their centres, often with little or contradictory information provided. This lack of information, insufficient access to cleaning supplies and PPE for some, and the inherent contradiction of providing care to young children while physical distancing combined to create high levels of anxiety around the risk of infection. Because of their low wages, lack of benefits, and limited sick pay, many educators did not have the power to refuse work they felt was unsafe. Those who did give up work did so at great personal cost. The risk that educators assumed conflicted with their ability to provide care to their own dependents, adding to their mental anguish.

Since this research was conducted, educators and their allies have continued to advocate for improvements in their sector, with the ongoing pandemic creating a policy window through which to effect change. As a result of this pressure, in March 2021 the federal government announced the Canada-Wide Early Learning and Child Care System, investing $30 billion over five years. Following an agreement between the British Columbia and federal governments, BC's March 2022 provincial budget dedicated $2.4 million in new child care spending and, importantly, announced its intention of bringing child care within the Ministry of Education. These developments, which hopefully will increase spaces, improve wages, and professionalize the sector, can be viewed as a silver lining to the pandemic. They are the direct result of educators' contributions and sacrifices in the initial months of the pandemic.

Educators offered recommendations on how such investments can be used to foster resilience in the sector. These include standardized health benefits, paid sick and care leave across the sector, increased wages, and public health training opportunities for educators. For future public health crises, they recommended that public health communication to childcare settings be streamlined through one channel and that childcare centres have access to government supply chains for PPE and cleaning materials, as well as on-site mental health support for educators and the children in their care. Most clearly, ECEs demanded that their voices be listened to and their expertise consulted as educators with direct experience and knowledge of the challenges of providing care during a pandemic.

8

Caring Too Much

Physicians

A colleague said to me "leave your heart at home." Women do get more emotionally involved, and it can be detrimental to our health. For those reasons it does put people off from stepping up to leadership roles.

Surgeon

In June 2020, just a few months into the pandemic, I received an email from a member of the Vancouver Coastal Health Physician Diversity, Equity and Inclusion Committee (DEI). She explained that the DEI committee and the Vancouver Physician Staff Association (VPSA) had decided to hold focus groups with women physicians to better understand their experiences during COVID-19. She asked if I would like to join and potentially use the findings within the Gender and COVID-19 research project. As a researcher, it is hard to say no to free data, especially data that aligned so clearly with my research interests, so I immediately said yes. I often think that if I had said, "No, I'm too busy" (I was working twelve-hour days and feeling incredibly guilty about not spending enough time with my kid), I might never have written this book. The focus groups that followed inspired the additional research with women frontline workers discussed in the previous chapters. I remain grateful to the physicians for the invitation and the inspiration.

Over the following year and a half, I have been surprised to see how little research focuses on the gender experiences of physicians during health crises. A literature review I contributed to found just one article (out of seventy-eight) on physicians, women, and health crises since 2010 (Morgan et al. 2022). This neglect may reflect the gender composition of medicine, which is the only sector within the health and social assistance field that remains male-dominated, with only 46 per cent of physicians identifying as women. Medicine is thus not "feminized" like the other sectors profiled in this book in compensation or working conditions. Physicians are comparatively well paid and enjoy high status both within the health system and Canadian society. While they are among those who serve "in the trenches," they are also the best resourced and have a high degree of autonomy.

This privilege sets women physicians apart from the other women whose experiences are recounted here, but it also makes gender analysis all the more crucial. Just as the feminized norms of the other professions already discussed shape those women's experiences, so do the masculine norms of medicine shape women physicians' work, income, and power. Women physicians continue to make less than men physicians, even within specialties, and medical leadership remains male-dominated (Cohen and Kiran 2020). The continued inequities in the field have been attributed to a combination of factors, including discriminatory hiring procedures, women physicians' unpaid care responsibilities, and metrics of success, such as research funding, that tend to favour men (Tricco et al. 2021). At the start of the pandemic, the associate editor of the *Journal of the American Medical Association*, Linda Brubaker (2020), predicted that COVID-19 would have dire effects on women physicians because the medical profession continues to be characterized by a "persistent life-work imbalance" that particularly disadvantages women. Similarly, Jones et al. (2020) discussed how the pandemic was increasing unpaid care work for women physicians, leading to reduced paid work. Both referred to the "double shift" of professional and care responsibilities that women physicians assume more often than men. As a result, despite their relative privilege, women physicians face similar challenges managing unpaid care and professional obligations, demonstrating that gender inequality affects all levels of society and all types of professions. Furthermore, during the pandemic, women physicians were not just battling a virus, but also the masculine norms and structures that shape their profession.

The DEI committee and VPSA held four focus groups: two in June 2020 (with eight physicians in one and six in the other) and two in September 2020 (with seven physicians in one and six in the other). Because the focus groups were originally conceived to bring women physicians together to share stories, support each other freely, and inform the advocacy efforts of the DEI committee and VPSA, they were not recorded. Instead, a member of the DEI committee and I took notes, which we later compared for accuracy. The focus groups were attended by physicians of a variety of backgrounds and specialties and included interactive polls, typed questions, and open discussions. Participants shared their personal and professional experiences, which I have tried to represent faithfully here, showing where their experiences converge and diverge. These focus groups were held during the first six months of the pandemic, so discussions of employment effects, burnout, and other challenges should be placed in that context.

THE QUADRUPLE BURDEN

The changes related to COVID-19 had varying effects on physicians' paid work, depending on their specialization. Some found that their work greatly increased due to new protocols and responsibilities. One physician explained, "There was a lot of fear we weren't going to have the proper PPE, that we wouldn't be able to protect ourselves. I was working sixty hours a week riddled with the anxiety around healthcare worker safety." Another described the first few weeks of the pandemic as "the hardest thing I've ever been through," and another noted, "[D]uring that first month and a half I didn't have time to think." An emergency room doctor noted that though fewer people came to the emergency room, because fear of infection or of overwhelming the health system kept many away, those who did come were often severely ill, injured, or "dead on arrival" – often because they had avoided earlier care out of a fear of COVID-19. At the other end of the continuum, family doctors experienced reduced demand. A general practitioner explained, "I felt useless. I wanted to do more, but I didn't know where I could go. As a community GP, we're on the front lines but our offices were stagnant for a while because patients wouldn't come. It was so slow."

Many took on extra responsibilities to make up for these feelings of futility. One physician explained, "I felt powerless as well. I used telehealth for doing my clinical work and did many webinars on any topic I could find – PPE, changes in protocols, COVID testing, etc. I wanted to do more too." Another noted, "I went into fight or flight. I did every webinar. I put my name into redeployment. I prepared to go into battle." The shift to virtual care required developing new skills on the fly, which many struggled with: "I was a late adopter with technology, then the pandemic changed things overnight. It was doable, but so much to learn. Things would be set up in the office and then have to be changed constantly based on recommendations ... it was so much change." Virtual care also blurred the boundaries between home and work, with participants describing "expectations are that one is on all of the time, checking and responding to emails constantly."

Shifts in workload affected all physicians, not just women, but for women this change was more often layered on top of their increased responsibilities at home. When asked, "[H]ave women physicians experienced the pandemic differently than men physicians?" twenty-two out of twenty-seven respondents said "yes, significantly different," or "yes, different," with five answering "slight difference" (see figure 8.1). When asked to explain this difference, many commented on the different approaches they took to COVID-19-related isolation to keep family members safe. One woman noted, "Male colleagues were better able to isolate for the week they were on COVID ward. Women wanted to isolate within [their] home because children are going to want their moms. Most of the women didn't feel they could up and leave." Another agreed, "I have young kids and not being able to isolate is a real concern for me." The physicians shared stories of men physicians isolating in hotels and rented apartments on their own, whereas women physicians camped out in their garages or yards.

The other common difference was related to who took responsibility for unpaid care work. One physician noted, "I was working from home through virtual care all throughout the pandemic. Between sessions, I would do housework, dishes, laundry, etc. Our life partners don't have to do that." Many women physicians found themselves responsible for a slew of household tasks they had previously outsourced: "Because I couldn't outsource, my housekeeper couldn't come, I had to do all of this. It was extremely frustrating how imbalanced it felt. It all came to me." In heterosexual couples, women were expected to resolve increased care burdens because "If the cleaner can't make it, the mom just ends up doing it all."

Physicians who were mothers in heterosexual relationships found that the responsibility to adapt to child care and school interruptions fell on them. One explained, "I have a young child at home and that has been the most challenging thing to deal with. The additional home responsibilities were daunting, and that was in addition to the

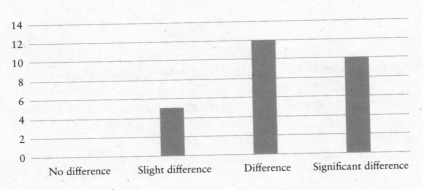

Figure 8.1 Focus group responses to poll question "Have women physicians experienced the pandemic differently than men physicians?"

precarious work situation." While physicians had access to child care for essential workers during the initial closures from March to June 2020, the challenge of making new arrangements was exacerbated by the lack of a coordinated emergency response within the childcare sector. As noted in chapter 7, it was up to providers to decide if they would continue to operate and at what capacity, and pre-COVID there was already an extreme shortage of child care, especially for parents doing shift work (Macdonald and Friendly 2021). Due to a dearth of childcare facilities and a lack of flexible options, many physicians had relied on nannies to provide in-home care. In the context of the uncertainty and fear of the early pandemic, many physicians agreed to lay off their nannies, who were concerned about the risk of infection because of physicians' high-risk profession, so that the nannies could access federal government unemployment benefits. The physician parents then had to seek out the facility-based child care provided for essential workers, which (despite being designated for healthcare workers doing shift work) had limited hours. One mother noted that her child's centre only provided care from 9 a.m. to 3 p.m., asking, "[W]ho works until 3 p.m.?"

Participants discussed why women were primarily responsible for unpaid care work. Numerous participants in multiple focus groups reiterated the feeling that "kids always want their mom." Women recognized that they also participated in perpetuating gender norms, and spoke of the challenge of delegating to others. One participant explained, "My husband provided child care when I was working; however, because I was in the house, I kept having the inclination to shorten my workday, or to intervene to help my husband to take care of our child." Another reflected, "I seem to need to be responsible for more things than men ... where does that come from?" Women physicians had internalized assumptions that they, as opposed to their partners, were responsible for unpaid care work and should be able to manage the double shift. When their previous coping mechanisms, such as outsourcing care work, were not available, they took on this responsibility and felt guilty when they struggled with it.

While such quotations position women physicians as imposing the responsibility for family care upon themselves, participants also noted that such assumptions are embedded in social and health systems. One physician explained that "with no child care available and both of us being essential workers, there was no consideration as to how this would be managed. The assumption is that I, as the mother, will stay home." Another physician mother recalled that even though the school also had the father's number, she was interrupted in the operating room by a call from her child's school because her child had developed possible COVID-19 symptoms. Another noted, "My kids had to isolate and were sent home. The school calls me at 1 p.m. and assumes that I should just go home and take care of the kids, even though my husband is far more flexible with his schedule. Why didn't they call him?" These women were somewhat befuddled by just how unequal the unpaid care burden was, despite their privilege and assumptions that gender equality prevailed in their homes and work environments. Not only was the unequal division of labour accepted within their families, but it was actively enforced by their employers, social systems, and even themselves. While their relative privilege shielded many women physicians from the multiple burdens placed on women during non-pandemic times, the crisis in care during COVID-19 reinforced unequal gender norms during a time that was also characterized by professional struggle.

BEING ESSENTIAL

Unlike some of the other professions recounted in this book, there was little ambiguity about whether physicians were considered essential. Most felt recognized as essential workers and appreciated signs of support such as food and other donations. They were privileged in their access to resources like PPE and sick pay. However, they still

experienced conflicts between their essential status and the lack of support for unpaid care work, which had notable financial implications.
One physician explained that, just that day, she had given up her shift
because her child had been sent home from school with COVID-19
symptoms. While physicians were provided with quarantine pay
through Doctors of BC if they had to miss work because of their own
COVID-19 exposure or infection, it was not provided if they could not
work because their kids had to isolate – an experience shared by many
focus group participants. Another physician noted that even when care
responsibilities were recognized, the financial conflict that care work
created for women physicians was not:

> In my department, it was expressed that if women wanted to
> take off time to take care of kids, people, meaning men, would
> take their call for them. People thought they were really well-
> meaning, and they were even evolved, that they were men of
> a new age that they were doing this. Then it was pointed out
> to them that they were just asking women, that they assumed
> women don't need an income.

This oversight obscured the fact that, in addition to being the primary
care providers in their families and essential workers, many women
physicians were also often the sole or primary income earners.

Physicians described "feeling mercenary talking about [loss of
income]. It's a stress most people won't talk about. Especially for
unpartnered physicians." Yet many women physicians were financially
affected by the drop in demand for services during the first few months
of the pandemic. Some specialists saw their services almost completely
shut down and spoke of their income going to zero overnight at the
same time that costs, such as child care, increased. One gynecologist
explained that since having children and dealing with some of her own
health issues, she had previously reduced her work hours. While this
financial decision had been viable at the time, COVID-19 made it
impossible: "I was working part time, doing fine. I gave up call last
year, so not much of my work could be done virtually when the restrictions were put in place. Not many patients were urgent, so I saw a
74 per cent decrease in income. $12,000 a month in overhead pay-
ments was very distressing. I didn't know how long this would last ...
I ended up closing my community practice last week." Not only were
women physicians more at risk of losing income because of unpaid

care responsibilities, but the gender wage gap meant they were also likely to be more vulnerable to the effects of reduced income (Mousa et al. 2021). Having an essential status, which only recognized their paid professional contribution to the response, did not protect them against such financial loss.

MENTAL HEALTH, MORAL DISTRESS, AND BURNOUT

Women physicians in BC described a context of "anticipation anxiety" and "pre-traumatic stress syndrome" in the early spring as they feared the pandemic would get worse – experiences that were common across genders (Kurt, Deveci, and Oguzoncul 2020). Surveys in other regions have found that women physicians, compared with men, reported higher rates of anxiety and depression during the pandemic (de Wit et al. 2020; Kurt, Deveci, and Oguzoncul 2020). Notably, when women spoke about their concerns, they did not separate professional and personal experiences. One physician explained that she hadn't eaten dinner with her two kids since the pandemic started: "I have guilt for not being with my family. The office staff is so dedicated, they sit there with me until I am done and miss time with their own families. They won't go home. There is guilt about that too. Everyone is doing fine, but we're starting to burn out." Another physician explained, "When COVID hit, I took a lot of work on and didn't think about my mental health. Now that the pandemic [has] slowed down, it has caught up to me, and in addition, my family members also suffered from health issues." Others described losing sleep worrying about colleagues, patients, and family members. One stated, "I was working around the clock (sixty hours per week), and the constant worry about other healthcare providers caused me to lose a lot of sleep." Another noted that working only from home had a negative effect, saying, "For me the pandemic meant isolation. I never met colleagues, no one ever asked once 'How are you doing?'" Physicians reported that declining mental wellness was widespread among their peers: "[I was] at a committee meeting with family physicians and a lot were getting very fatigued and almost burnt out, if not burnt out, particularly the ones with children," and "I've seen others juggling family life, virtual care, then more things are opening up, it's scary. Requirements keep changing, people are fatigued."

Physicians who were working with populations particularly at risk of adverse health outcomes related to COVID-19 experienced

acute levels of stress. One physician who worked in the LTC
sector explained:

> Working with older adults, the frail[est] of the frail and the fact
> that they could be harmed by being in contact with me was a
> source of anxiety to me. Also, transitioning to work from home
> was difficult. Getting used to the new technology and helping
> the patients who are often elderly who didn't know how to
> use the technology was challenging. The elderly patients had
> hearing or vision issues that made explaining to them the use
> of technology challenging.

She felt very anxious about potentially transmitting COVID-19 to this
vulnerable population: "My work involves visiting nursing homes.
I still get anxious about sharing the virus when going into people's
homes. I get tested even with a sniffle. This feels like a smaller challenge compared to the stress of others." She was also exposed to the
trauma that residents and staff in LTC facilities were experiencing
(described in chapter 2), saying, "I can see the effect on seniors, who
are isolated, have less resources and support available to them now
than before (community/social resources). There is stress for families,
worrying about their family members in nursing homes, alone, the
threat of outbreak, etc. There have been more deaths. Staff have had
to talk to families. There is a lot of stress and trauma that has affected
the staff."

Many physicians experienced similar anxiety in their role as primary care providers to older parents. One noted, "Initially, there
was a lot of effort invested in restructuring how we do our clinical work. That, coupled with constant worry about elder parents
who were ill during a time when the elderly were most at risk, was
challenging and a source of anxiety." Many expressed their fear of
transmitting COVID-19 to family members: "You're not just worried
about yourself, but if you're going to give it to others, like elderly
parents" and "then you're worried about the parents. So, you're
kind of stuck in the middle. There is this ongoing stress that you just
don't expect." Some had taken measures to distance themselves from
older family members, but this was replaced by guilt about unfulfilled
care responsibilities: "My parents are in their 80s. Not being able
to see them in person and make sure they're OK, I had a lot of anxiety
about them."

POWER

Leadership within health systems, and particularly among physicians, remains male-dominated. This is explained partly by the barriers women face in taking on leadership responsibilities, such as lack of time due to unpaid care work, and by the type of leadership qualities prized in the profession. Within the field, leadership traits more often associated with men (for example, traits used more frequently in reference letters for male physicians), such as assertiveness, are often valued over those most often associated with women, such as being collaborative (Trix and Psenka 2016; Turrentine et al. 2019). Whether men are actually more assertive and women more collaborative is another debate, since expectations can influence how men and women are perceived and what type of leadership is valued.

Women's inadequate representatation in leadership positions has been shown, in other contexts, to result in policies that do not take gender inequality or women's specific needs into account (Mooi-Reci and Risman 2021). Many of the women physicians who participated in the focus groups felt that decision-makers, who were primarily men and did not have unpaid care responsibilities, did not recognize the challenges they faced: "Male leaders were making decisions that had to be made quickly, but [they] also had a stay-at-home wife or children who were no longer dependent on them." Many participants noted that changes in scheduling because of the COVID-19 response did not take unpaid care responsibilities into consideration, with one participant noting, "[T]hey assume there is this model where there is someone to look after kids." Women physicians felt that decision-makers, who assumed physicians had the choice to prioritize one or the other, did not recognize their need to both work and care for their family.

This lack of consideration was exacerbated by what participants described as a "command and control" approach during the first few months of the pandemic: "Men are making more decisions now with less process or consultation, they are more directive and dictatorial. Men are advancing their careers and using a more command-and-control style." While it was recognized that decisions often had to be made rapidly in the context of an unfolding emergency, lack of consultation also made decision-making more exclusive: "Men have become more directive. They're using COVID to avoid consultation. They seem to just proceed and decide." Some physicians felt that the COVID-19 response included a return to patriarchal attitudes, describing increased instances of sexist comments and talking down to women: "The old-school, traditional male traits became very prominent during this time. Men in leadership roles become more intolerant and abusive verbally, and overall difficult to deal with." One participant felt that such behaviour reflected unhealthy expressions of stress: "Because everyone was stressed, everyone was anxious, I saw a regression to intolerance. Old-school man behaviour was heightened during COVID, the mansplaining, the talking down to women." Another felt the emergency response was used to excuse such behaviour: "[COVID] allowed people to just assume and make statements like that. They felt like this before but now it's OK to say." Such behaviour did not affect just women but also younger men and physicians from ethnic and racial minorities. Such abuse discouraged some women from participating in decision-making. A woman physician of South Asian descent said the increased sexism and racism "has affected me emotionally that a lot of that abuse was turned towards me, to the extent that I didn't want to attend meetings with those leaders any longer." Within the initial emergency response, the "tyranny of the urgent" led to consultation and equity processes being de-prioritized, resulting in women physicians feeling unrepresented and, at times, abused by male-dominated leadership (Smith 2019).

Many focus group participants perceived the women leaders who had stepped up during COVID-19 as more consultative and caring. One participant explained, "Where men's decision-making has been dictatorial, women reach out more, bring people together, reach consensus, while managing multiple responsibilities." Participants reported receiving encouragement and support from women leaders who, despite the urgency of the emergency response, took time to ask about their mental health, wellness, and family life: "I had to work from home, and the response of my female colleagues in leadership roles was more compassionate and supportive during this time. Women leaders tended to ask more '[H]ow are you today?' and 'How are things at home?'" Another woman reflected that "A non-physician woman manager sent out an email telling everyone to give themselves a break and take some time off – being reminded of that has helped." Previous research has found that women physicians in Canada felt greater competence in non-verbal communication and handling sensitive issues than their male counterparts during patient interactions (Lovell, Lee, and Brotheridge 2009); the results here suggest that they also employ these skills in interactions with their peers.

The perception of women leaders as more caring than men may also reflect personal internalized gender bias, in that women physicians are more likely than men to be described with related terms, such as compassionate, but participants' examples suggest that such perceptions were also based on personal experiences (Carnes et al. 2015). This then raises questions about whether women fulfill more "caring" leadership roles because of internalized stereotypes (they feel it is expected of them), or to fill a gap that is not being met by other leaders, or for other and combined reasons. The women who participated in the focus groups described taking on leadership roles because they wanted to contribute to the COVID-19 response and out of concern for colleagues, particularly those they saw struggling with child care and elder-care responsibilities, suggesting they were responding to an identified need.

However, instead of being rewarded for taking on caring leadership roles, women often felt censured: "A colleague said to me '[L]eave your heart at home.' Women do get more emotionally involved, and it can be detrimental to our health. For those reasons it does put people off from stepping up to leadership roles." Participants spoke of feeling overburdened by the need to support others during the crisis and having the sense that their emotional labour was undervalued: "I am told that 'I care too much.' And it's true, I care ... I don't know if I will be able to continue to be a leader for too long. The mental well-being toll is great." While other women spoke with appreciation of women leaders who took time to care for others, and such leadership is celebrated in the health literature (Mousa et al. 2021), there was a perception that it was not valued overall within the health system. Such devaluing reflects stereotypes about what type of leadership is celebrated (e.g., authoritative, decisive, and rational, as opposed to collaborative, caring, and emotional) within the medical field in general and during a crisis response in particular. Caring was positioned as a personal liability rather than an asset among physicians in the COVID-19 response.

While women leaders felt critiqued for "caring too much," some also felt they were not given credit for their formal professional contributions. One participant recounted being assigned to compile some documentation early in the outbreak, but when it came time to present, men physicians got credit for her work. Another responded, "I echo the experience of seeing women doing the work and men taking the credit. Usually through having a leadership position and presenting the work." Others noted, "Seems men have the face time of the department, yet women do the work behind the scenes."

Despite these attitudes, many women physicians had taken on greater leadership roles, recognizing a need for their skills and presence in decision-making. One participant argued, "I think that the pandemic has created an opportunity to help women to move into leadership roles and help develop new leaders." A number noted that the presence of women leaders at the provincial and national levels had inspired more women to step up: "The leaders of the COVID response have in many cases been predominantly women. Watching them, I decided to join a meeting to learn how to become a better leader, and to find out how I can learn about leadership skills." Others felt that the shift toward more virtual work made it easier to take on leadership roles. Women could attend meetings and conferences virtually, reducing travel times and childcare challenges: "It feels like a new phase of life, where things can be done differently, and people have to find new ways to become a leader. It has given me faith that maybe it can be done without all the expectations for putting in face time, conferences, etc." Such faith was spread through increased virtual peer support networks, "The silver lining of this pandemic was that it has created opportunities for collegiality – many virtual groups were set up across the country and this has encouraged women to interact with each other and support each other. Predominantly, women joined these groups."

CONCLUSION

In June 2020, one of the focus group participants described telling her clinic staff, who were working late with her once again, "Don't worry, in September, things will be better." In September 2020, a participant noted, "When you say six months [since the start of the pandemic], I feel like I've been doing this for three years." I reflect on these quotes in March 2022, and these women are still on the front lines at home and at work. The focus group participants' perspectives demonstrate that they never simply experienced the initial months of the pandemic as physicians; they lived them as women with increased care responsibilities both outside of the formal health systems and the limited opportunities within it. Pre-pandemic assumptions within families and communities that women would absorb private care deficits at their own cost and the lack of supportive health systems shaped women physicians' multiple burdens. Their experiences show that unpaid care work at home and emotional labour at work are determinants of poor mental health, exacerbated by a lack of recognition and support within health systems.

Women physicians offered ideas on how to support their empowerment. They ranged from having flexible childcare options on-site to intentionally inclusive leadership structures and leadership training specifically for women. They also felt that mental health supports need to be provided within hospital settings, including those targeted at men who expressed stress in harmful ways. As one participant put it, "We all need psychological PPE."

9

We've Been through a Heck of a Thing

Conclusion

Trauma can you lead you to [a] place of burnout, stress, and mental health disorder. Or with early intervention, it can lead you to a place of increased resilience. And what path we go down for each individual is not going to be determined by their own individual circumstances but by what supports we put in place for that person ... Because we've been through a heck of a thing and if we can come out on the other end relatively whole, then that gives us more confidence in your own abilities going forward to handle really challenging situations.

Long-term-care manager

Each group of women included in this book can be viewed as a branch of a defence force with slightly different purposes but engaged in the same conflict. Women working in LTC were in the trenches of the response, the most likely to come face-to-face with the virus, saving the lives of those most vulnerable. Nurses provided direct care not only to COVID-19 patients but also to bystanders afflicted by the secondary health effects of the pandemic. The home front was staffed by teachers, early childhood educators, and moms attempting to maintain a sense of normalcy while providing the care work that enabled other essential workers to fulfill their roles. Midwives were the resistance, working in the shadows, but still essential. Physicians had privileged positions, similar to those of officers in the military, but, because of that, also had to contend with masculine systems of command and control.

In many ways, again like soldiers sent into a violent conflict, these women were set up to fail. The predominance of outbreaks in LTC was due not only to COVID-19's severe effects on the older population but to the historical neglect of the sector, located as it was at the periphery of the health system, often as for-profit businesses, and inadequately resourced and staffed at the best of times. This understaffing meant that when the crisis hit, many residents went without basic necessities such as baths, and workers experienced second-hand trauma. Without guaranteed access to even the most basic PPE, midwives were unable do their jobs safely, putting the health of new parents and infants at risk. Greater care responsibilities were thrust on mothers in a context of reduced support, particularly where the needs were the greatest. Children with special needs became ill because their parents did not receive adequate support. Lack of child care caused doctors to miss shifts, affecting patient care. Despite such scenarios, these women rose to the challenge, donning their "thick mom skin" like battle armour, going above and beyond to provide care to those most isolated and in need. The limits they came up against were not of their own making, but the result of systemic inequities and policy choices made both before and during the crisis.

Gendered frontline experience contrasts with the celebration of Canada's and BC's GBA+ approach to pandemic response. While significant investments have been made to address flagship gendered issues, such as child care and IPV, no action is being taken to address broader political and economic structures, such as working conditions in the care economy. The federal and provincial approaches of providing resources to individuals (ranging from CERB payments to virtual mental health services) provided some immediate relief but failed to address the structural determinants (such as lack of access to child care, housing, and justice) of the worst effects of the pandemic on women and essential workers. The dominant neoliberal paradigm guiding the Canadian government's approaches to gender inequality placed responsibility on the individual, without recognizing that their unequal access to resources limited women's ability to seize those opportunities (Paterson 2010). As a result, pandemic pay top-ups or token recognition did not overcome the legacy of inadequate investments in the care infrastructure. Increasing salaries in the LTC sector did not attract enough new staff to address chronic shortages. Posters of superheroes in hospitals did not ensure that nurses and midwives had access to PPE. While demonstrating resourcefulness, even the many strategies women employed to overcome the challenges and effects of frontline work, such as connecting with peers and professional development, still reflect individualistic responses to social-structural challenges and so were limited in their effectiveness.

As a result, the challenges frontline workers experienced during COVID-19 will have long-term effects for healthcare and education systems in Canada. Faith in the ability of the current LTC system to provide adequate and safe, never mind compassionate, care has been, rightly, shaken. Human resources (i.e., the women included in this book) are depleted, with both the BC Nurses Union (2021) and the Hospital Employees' Union (2022) reporting that over a third of their members are thinking of leaving healthcare work. Interruptions in schooling and early childhood education are projected to have negative effects on children's development (Haeck and Larose 2022). Youth are experiencing mental health crises because of the disruptions in their education and home life (Hawke et al. 2021). These system- and society-level impacts are the cumulative effects of inadequate investments in the care economy and the people who keep it going.

Just as the long-term consequences will reverberate within health and education systems for years to come, they will be lived by women like those represented here who have sacrificed career and training opportunities to fill elder-care and childcare gaps. There is a real risk that women whose careers were interrupted by care responsibilities during COVID-19 will experience penalties in promotions and advancement, much like the motherhood penalty associated with taking parental leave. Equally concerning is the potential long-term effect on women's health, considering the trauma, moral distress, and sustained anxiety frontline workers have experienced. Healthcare workers are already describing the ongoing effects of PTSD on their work, as well as their home life and health (d'Ettorre et al. 2021). If both the systems- and individual-level long-term effects, which are intrinsically linked to each other, are to be mitigated, we must learn from the experiences of women on the front lines.

THE QUADRUPLE BURDEN

A key lesson is to recognize that the women whose experiences are shared here fulfilled more than one essential role: caring for patients, older adults, and/or children during both their paid time and their unpaid time. These roles cannot be separated, but directly affected each other, with increased burdens in one aspect of work reducing time or energy for the others. Care, while hard to quantify, is not an infinite resource. It takes time, supplies, and energy, and when these run out, those responsible for care must make up the shortfall at their own cost, or at the cost of those they provide care to. The experiences included here also demonstrate that care work during COVID entailed more than physical care. Midwives did not just check for a fetal heart rate; they eased new and expectant parents' anxiety at a time of great uncertainty. Teachers did not just educate children; they answered questions from anxious parents and provided emotional support to their peers. LTC workers didn't just do their regular work; they facilitated connections between family and residents. Notably, many women described these additional and emotional-labour roles as originally drawing them to their profession, providing the rewards they valued, though in a context with little material benefit. However, as their multiple burdens grew and became prolonged, and their ability to connect became more fraught, these rewards decreased and instead became burdens. Care work – both paid and unpaid – can be fulfilling and meaningful, even or especially during a crisis, but only when it is appropriately resourced and recognized.

BEING ESSENTIAL

The COVID-19 pandemic has reinforced arguments long made by feminist philosophers and feminist political economists about the importance, or essential nature, of care work to societal and economic development (Larrabee 2016; Folbre, Gautham, and Smith 2021; Rai and Waylen 2013). As communities and health and education systems faced an unprecedented threat, the care work provided mostly by women was called upon to maintain order and ensure basic needs were met. While many of the professions here were celebrated as essential, this label exposed contradictions more often than it contributed to empowering women. Physicians noted that despite being essential, they did not have access to child care when they needed it. Meanwhile, childcare workers did not have input into how their sector responded to the pandemic. Nurses described the dissonance between hero-worshipping public relations statements and their lack of access to simple items like coffee and bathroom breaks. Essential status did not translate into teachers being prioritized for vaccines. As a result, being labelled essential rarely resulted in these women being empowered; instead, it created a demand that they continue to fill these roles regardless of declining work conditions and supports. Recognition of the centrality of the care economy remained limited to celebrating roles that sustained the current order as opposed to challenging it (Folbre, Gautham, and Smith 2021).

Such limitations were further made evident by which roles were recognized as essential and which were not. Midwifery and mothering, both of which ensure child and mother well-being, were not formally recognized as essential. Childcare educators, who provided the first layer of care, enabling other care providers to do their essential work, felt under-recognized. The lack of formal recognition of the importance of child care, whether provided by mothers or educators, is nothing new, but it is notable that even during a crisis that exponentially increased this work and clearly demonstrated its centrality to economic functioning, this willful ignorance persisted. Such differences support midwives' assertions that the marginalization of their profession reflects a de-prioritization of the health of women and children in general and suggest that this hierarchy extends throughout the care sector.

MENTAL HEALTH, MORAL DISTRESS, AND BURNOUT

All the women who participated in this research reported heightened stress and anxiety from the conflict between their desire to provide quality care while maintaining physical distance and the fear of infecting those they cared for at work and at home. The inability to meet standards of care led to moral distress, which contributed to burnout. Many of these effects, while linked to the pandemic, could have been prevented and mitigated. While it is rarely possible to eradicate the direct cause of moral distress (such as the pandemic), it is possible to rectify its secondary effects, such as workers not having a voice in decision-making or being understaffed (Pauly, Varcoe, and Storch 2012). For example, child care that corresponds to shift work and includes services for children with special needs could have eased moral distress related to mothering. Having public health professionals do contact tracing would have enabled school leaders to get some sleep. Adequate staffing in LTC would have prevented workers from having to decide who got a bath that week and who had to go without. In-person therapy could have enabled nurses who had witnessed

COVID-19-related deaths to process their grief. Women in need knew that phone calls to a mental health hotline would not increase resident-to-staff ratios, and moms with toddlers underfoot didn't have the time or privacy for virtual counselling sessions – so they rarely accessed these services. Instead, they turned to "cocktails of Benadryl and wine" or, when possible, peer support.

POWER

In response to the negative effects of COVID-19 on their health and well-being, women advocated for change in both very immediate and sustained ways. Childcare educators insisted that their safety was just as important as that of the parents of the children they cared for. Midwives succeeded in gaining access to the PPE provided to other frontline healthcare workers. Nurses asserted that their lived experiences provided expertise that was just as valid alongside scientific research. Teachers and physicians seized the opportunity of online learning to advance their credentials and careers. Despite exhaustion, multiple responsibilities, and inadequate resources, women fought for their basic rights and for those to whom they provided care.

Transforming these inequities at all levels will require grappling with dominant, often unseen, forms of oppression. The accounts included here demonstrate how the "tyranny of the urgent" prevailed to restrict women's participation in leadership, entrenching top-down decision-making structures that became even less accessible to women during the crisis (Smith 2019). The leadership justified their command-and-control responses by the emergency nature of the initial response, supposedly necessitating quick decision-making based on technical and scientific approaches, as opposed to experiential and emotional knowledge. The result was to prevent women from being able to make more compassionate decisions that were informed by their lived experience. Educators' requests to temporarily close childcare facilities were denied. Women physicians were dismissed as "too caring." LTC workers were made to fear punishment for not following protocols rather than being asked for input into how they could be improved. Across all sectors, women felt that their leadership contributions were often overlooked or co-opted, and that the emotional support they provided was undervalued. Being unequally represented in leadership before the outbreak and not consulted during it, combined with the time limits imposed by the double shift (of paid and unpaid work), reduced women's opportunities to communicate with leadership and respond to the challenges they faced, entrenching masculine bias in the decisions that were made during the pandemic.

Impediments to participating in leadership decisions not only disempowered and discouraged women essential workers but also impeded the effectiveness of the overall response to COVID-19. Teachers' expertise as parents was not incorporated into school planning. Nurses' personal experiences of risk did not inform PPE policies. The gap in healthcare protocols in childcare settings could have been filled by combining educators' knowledge of their sector with public health expertise. Previous research has emphasized the importance of women in decision-making bodies (Downs et al. 2014). The experiences here further suggest that much expertise is lost by not engaging and consulting with the women who have the most intimate knowledge of the pandemic – those on the front lines.

The barriers to women's participation in leading a pandemic response they staffed demonstrate an urgent need for organizations to intervene to develop health, education, and care systems that support women (Mousa et al. 2021). Their shared experience of the pandemic, as well as their common struggles and goals, suggests that there is an opportunity to create coalitions across sectors so that women essential workers can advocate for greater gender equality (Folbre, Gautham, and Smith 2021). Midwives' descriptions of how other health professionals supported them in accessing PPE and descriptions of positive peer support among essential workers suggest that there is already a movement toward forms of mutual empowerment among women. Such efforts might capitalize on mobilizing nationally and globally to invest in care infrastructure and calls for more representative health leadership (UN Women 2021).

LOOKING FORWARD

Tricco et al. (2021) write, of advancing gender equity within health systems, "Multipronged interventions composed of a combination of structural and individual interventions ... are needed to foster lasting and meaningful change ... solutions must begin with recognition of the systemic nature of the problem." The federal and BC governments have taken some notable, if limited, steps in this direction. The federal government's "feminist" budgets in particular have included increased funding for organizations addressing IPV and non-profits initiating gender equity–related projects. These investments have the potential to address many of the determinants of women's personal and economic security. For example, unprecedented investments in child care will ease unpaid-care burdens borne by mothers. However, such gains remain limited, with the effects on childcare educators less clear, since calls for a provincial wage grid and other efforts to improve working conditions have not, as of March 2022, been heeded (CCCABC 2022). The continued focus on working mothers rather than those providing paid child care suggests a continued approach of downloading care work without recognizing who is doing it or the value of their labour to broader social and economic development. Reflecting further incremental reform, efforts are underway to improve the LTC sector, with some workers, such as those in housekeeping and food service, moving back "in-house" instead of being contracted out (HEU 2021). This is expected to improve working conditions and wages, as is growing union membership. However, advocates are still calling for a shift away from private, for-profit care and greater investment in the health-care workforce more generally (Office of the Seniors Advocate 2021). Because these calls are occurring in a context of continued economic uncertainty and rising inflation, as well as counter-calls to reduce government spending, there is a real threat that care workers already on the point of burnout will be asked to continue much as they have been. There is a need to truly commit to developing a caring democracy in Canada that recognizes care as the centre of our lives and democratic political life (Tronto 2013)

Many of the recommendations from women on how to improve pandemic recovery and preparedness were similar across occupation groups, indicating opportunities to combine forces to agitate for transformation. All participants identified the need for more accessible child care, with those doing shift work emphasizing the need for child care that meshed with their schedules. Staffing shortages were a common theme, as was the need for employers to recognize women's multiple care responsibilities, allowing them greater flexibility and support. Most commented on the importance of active rather than passive mental health interventions, preferably at the worksite and accessible during paid time. Paid sick days were also required not only for essential workers but also for the care of dependents. All agreed that in the case of an outbreak, decisions about PPE should be made by those providing frontline care to patients. One-off cash transfers and tokens of appreciation were less helpful, but time for self-care was greatly appreciated. The definition of essential services during a crisis must consider those who are made most vulnerable, such as those with special needs, newcomers, and those fleeing violence. There was also a clear message about reforming approaches to emergency management to ensure that women and equity-deserving groups are meaningfully involved in making decisions. These recommendations can serve as a map for the way forward, not only for pandemic recovery but toward more just and equitable systems of care. Based on conversations with over 200 women working on the front lines, I am confident they would much prefer such reforms to any tokens or ceremonies of heroism.

References

Abrams, Elissa M., and Stanley J. Szefler. 2020. "COVID-19 and the Impact of Social Determinants of Health." *The Lancet Respiratory Medicine* 8, no. 7: 659–61. https://doi.org/10.1016/S2213-2600(20)30234-4.

Allen, Rebecca, John Jerrim, and Sam Sims. 2020. *How did the Early Stages of the COVID-19 Pandemic affect Teacher Wellbeing?* Centre for Education Policy and Equalising Opportunities. https://repec-cepeo.ucl.ac.uk/cepeow/old-style/cepeowp20-15.pdf.

Antonopoulos, Rania. 2008. "The Unpaid Care Work-Paid Work Connection." Annadale-on-Hudson: Levy Economics Institute, Bard College. http://www.levyinstitute.org.

ATA. 2020. "Teacher Pandemic Pulse Survey Results 2020–2021." Alberta Teachers' Association. https://legacy.teachers.ab.ca/COVID-19/2020-School-Re-entry/Pages/Teacher-Pandemic-Pulse-Survey-Results--Fall-2020.aspx.

– 2022. "Teacher Pandemic Pulse Survey Results: Spring, Fall and Winter 2020–2022." Alberta Teachers' Association. https://legacy.teachers.ab.ca/COVID-19/2020-School-Re-entry/Pages/Teacher-Pandemic-Pulse-Survey-Results--Fall-2020.aspx.

Badone, Ellen. 2021. "From Cruddiness to Catastrophe: COVID-19 and Long-Term Care in Ontario." *Medical Anthropology* 40, no. 5: 389–403. https://doi.org/10.1080/01459740.2021.1927023.

Baier, Annette C. 1985. "What Do Women Want in a Moral Theory?" *Noûs* 19, no. 1: 53–63. https://doi.org/10.2307/2215117.

BC Care Providers Association. 2019. "Filling the Gap." Vancouver: BC Care Providers Association. https://bccare.ca/wp-content/uploads/2019/03/Filling-the-Gap-March-2019.pdf.

BC Coroners Service. 2021. "Statistical Reports on Deaths in British
    Columbia – Province of British Columbia." Victoria: Government
    of British Columbia. https://www2.gov.bc.ca/gov/content/life-events/
    death/coroners-service/statistical-reports.

BCNU. 2021. "The Future of Nursing in BC." Victoria: BC Nurses Union.
    www.bcnu.org.

BCWHF. 2020. "Unmasking Gender Inequity." Vancouver: BC Women's
    Health Foundation. https://www.unmaskgenderinequity.ca.

Beauvoir, Simone de. 1949. *The Second Sex*. Translated by Constance
    Borde and Sheila Malovany-Chevallier. New York: Penguin Random
    House. 800.

Bennett, Dean. 2021. "Alberta Social Studies Plan Raises Questions on
    History, Religion, First Nations." *Toronto Star,* 30 March 2021. https://
    www.thestar.com/news/canada/2021/03/30/alberta-social-studies-plan-
    raises-questions-on-history-religion-first-nations.html.

Benoit, Cecilia, Sirpa Wrede, Ivy Bourgeault, Jane Sandall, Raymond de
    Vries, and Edwin R. van Teijlingen. 2005. "Understanding the Social
    Organisation of Maternity Care Systems: Midwifery as a Touchstone."
    Sociology of Health & Illness 27, no. 6: 722–37. https://doi.
    org/10.1111/J.1467-9566.2005.00471.X.

Berry, Isha, Jean Paul R. Soucy, Ashleigh Tuite, and David Fisman. 2020.
    "Open Access Epidemiologic Data and an Interactive Dashboard to
    Monitor the COVID-19 Outbreak in Canada." *CMAJ* 192, no. 5: E420.
    https://doi.org/10.1503/CMAJ.75262.

Braedley, Susan, and Meg Luxton. 2021. "Social Reproduction at Work,
    Social Reproduction as Work: A Feminist Political Economy Perspective."
    Journal of Labor and Society 1:1–28. https://doi.org/10.1163/
    24714607-BJA10049.

Brassolotto, Julia, Tamara Daly, Pat Armstrong, and Vishaya Naidoo.
    2017. "Experiences of Moral Distress by Privately Hired Companions
    in Ontario's Long-Term Care Facilities." *Quality in Ageing and
    Older Adults* 18, no. 1: 58–68. https://doi.org/10.1108/QAOA-12-
    2015-0054.

Braun, Virginia, and Victoria Clarke. 2014. "What Can 'Thematic
    Analysis' Offer Health and Wellbeing Researchers?" *International
    Journal of Qualitative Studies on Health and Well-Being* 9, no. 1.
    https://doi.org/10.3402/QHW.V9.26152.

Brubaker, Linda. 2020. "Women Physicians and the COVID-19
    Pandemic." *JAMA – Journal of the American Medical Association* 324,
    no. 9: 835–6. https://doi.org/10.1001/jama.2020.14797.

Bryson, Valerie, and Ruth Deery. 2010. "Public Policy, 'Men's Time' and Power: The Work of Community Midwives in the British National Health Service." *Women's Studies International Forum* 33, no. 2: 91–8. https://doi.org/10.1016/J.WSIF.2009.11.004.

Butler, Judith. 2020. "Performative Acts and Gender Constitution: An Essay in Phenomenology and Feminist Theory." In *Feminist Theory Reader: Local and Global Perspectives*, 5th ed., edited by Carole R. McCann, Seung-kyung Kim, and Emek Ergun, 353–61. London: Routledge. https://doi.org/10.4324/9781003001201-42.

Cameron, Anna, and Lindsay Tedds. 2020. "Gender-Based Analysis Plus (GBA+) and Intersectionality: Overview, an Enhanced Framework, and a British Columbia Case Study." *Social Science Research Network*, 1 December 2020. https://ssrn.com/abstract=3781905.

CARE Canada. 2020. "Canada Leads 30 Countries in Gender-Responsive COVID Action: New Report Highlights Room for Improvement in Humanitarian Response." Toronto: Care Canada. https://care.ca/wp-content/uploads/2020/06/CARE_COVID-19-womens-leadership-report_June-2020.2.pdf.

Carnes, Molly, Christie M. Bartels, Anna Kaatz, and Christine Kolehmainen. 2015. "Why Is John More Likely to Become Department Chair than Jennifer?" *Transactions of the American Clinical and Climatological Association* 126: 197–214. https://www.ncbi.nlm.nih.gov/pmc/articles/PMC4530686.

CCCABC. 2022. "2022 Budget Submission." Vancouver: Coalition of Child Care Advocates of BC. https://www.cccabc.bc.ca/2022_budget_submission.

Cecco, Leyland. 2020. "Canada: Neglected Residents and Rotten Food Found at Care Homes Hit by Covid-19." *Guardian*, 26 May 2020. https://www.theguardian.com/world/2020/may/26/canada-care-homes-military-report-coronavirus.

Chatelier, Stephen, and Sophie Rudolph. 2018. "Teacher Responsibility: Shifting Care from Student to (Professional) Self?" *British Journal of Sociology of Education* 39, no. 1: 1–15. https://doi.org/10.1080/01425692.2017.1291328.

Christoffersen, Ashlee, and Olena Hankivsky. 2021. "Responding to Inequities in Public Policy: Is GBA+ the Right Way to Operationalize Intersectionality?" *Canadian Public Administration* 64, no. 3: 524–31. https://doi.org/10.1111/CAPA.12429.

Ciciolla, Lucia, and Suniya S. Luthar. 2019. "Invisible Household Labor and Ramifications for Adjustment: Mothers as Captains of Households."

Sex Roles 81, no. 7–8: 467–86. https://doi.org/10.1007/S11199-018-1001-X/TABLES/7.

CIHI. 2021a. "COVID-19 Cases and Deaths in Health Care Workers in Canada." Ottawa: Canadian Institute for Health Information. https://www.cihi.ca/en/covid-19-cases-and-deaths-in-health-care-workers-in-canada.

– 2021b. "The Impact of COVID-19 on Long-Term Care in Canada: Focus on the First 6 Months." Ottawa: Canadian Institute for Health Information. https://www.cihi.ca/sites/default/files/document/impact-covid-19-long-term-care-canada-first-6-months-report-en.pdf.

CMHA. 2020. "Summary of Findings Mental Health Impacts of COVID-19: Wave 2." Vancouver: Canadian Mental Health Association. https://cmha.ca/wp-content/uploads/2020/12/CMHA-UBC-wave-2-Summary-of-Findings-FINAL-EN.pdf.

Cohen, Michelle, and Tara Kiran. 2020. "Closing the Gender Pay Gap in Canadian Medicine." *CMAJ* 192, no. 35: E1011–17. https://doi.org/10.1503/cmaj.200375.

Cohn, Carol. 1987. "Sex and Death in the Rational World of Defense Intellectuals on JSTOR." *Within and Without: Women, Gender, and Theory* 12, no. 4: 687–718. https://www.jstor.org/stable/3174209.

Collins, Caitlyn, Liana Christin Landivar, Leah Ruppanner, and William J. Scarborough. 2020. "COVID-19 and the Gender Gap in Work Hours." *Gender, Work and Organization* 28, no. S1: 101–12. https://doi.org/10.1111/gwao.12506.

Curran, Melissa A., Brandon T. McDaniel, Amanda M. Pollitt, and Casey J. Totenhagen. 2015. "Gender, Emotion Work, and Relationship Quality: A Daily Diary Study." *Sex Roles* 73, no. 3–4: 157–73. https://doi.org/10.1007/S11199-015-0495-8/TABLES/3.

Davies, Sara E., and Belinda Bennett. 2016. "A Gendered Human Rights Analysis of Ebola and Zika: Locating Gender in Global Health Emergencies." *International Affairs* 92, no. 5: 1041–60. https://doi.org/10.1111/1468-2346.12704.

Davies, Sara E., Sophie Harman, Rashida Manjoo, Maria Tanyag, and Clare Wenham. 2019. "Why It Must Be a Feminist Global Health Agenda." *The Lancet* 393, no. 10171: 601–3. https://doi.org/10.1016/S0140-6736(18)32472-3.

Daya, Rumina, and Jon Azpiri. 2020. "Calls to Vancouver Domestic-Violence Crisis Line Spike 300% amid COVID-19 Pandemic." *Global News*, 7 April 2020. https://globalnews.ca/news/6789403/domestic-violence-coronavirus.

Dean, Liz, Brendan Churchill, and Leah Ruppanner. 2022. "The Mental Load: Building a Deeper Theoretical Understanding of How Cognitive and Emotional Labor Overload Women and Mothers." *Community, Work and Family* 25, no. 1: 13–29. https://doi.org/10.1080/13668803.2021.2002813.

d'Ettorre, Gabriele, Giancarlo Ceccarelli, Letizia Santinelli, Paolo Vassalini, Giuseppe Pietro Innocenti, Francesco Alessandri, Alexia E. Koukopoulos, Alessandro Russo, Gabriella d'Ettorre, and Lorenzo Tarsitani. 2021. "Post-Traumatic Stress Symptoms in Healthcare Workers Dealing with the COVID-19 Pandemic: A Systematic Review." *International Journal of Environmental Research and Public Health* 18, no. 2: 601. https://doi.org/10.3390/ijerph18020601

de Wit, Kerstin, Mathew Mercuri, Clare Wallner, Natasha Clayton, Patrick Archambault, Kerri Ritchie, Caroline Gérin-Lajoie, Sara Gray, Lisa Schwartz, and Teresa Chan. 2020. "Canadian Emergency Physician Psychological Distress and Burnout during the First 10 Weeks of COVID-19: A Mixed-Methods Study." *Journal of the American College of Emergency Physicians Open* 1, no. 5: 1030–8. https://doi.org/10.1002/emp2.12225.

D'Ignazio, Catherine, and Lauren Klein. 2020. *Data Feminism*. Cambridge: MIT Press.

Downs, Jennifer A., Lindsey K. Reif, Adolfine Hokororo, and Daniel W. Fitzgerald. 2014. "Increasing Women in Leadership in Global Health." *Academic Medicine* 89, no. 8: 1103–7. https://doi.org/10.1097/ACM.0000000000000369.

Duan, Yinfei, Ala Iaconi, Yuting Song, Peter G. Norton, Janet E. Squires, Janice Keefe, Greta G. Cummings, and Carole A. Estabrooks. 2020. "Care Aides Working Multiple Jobs: Considerations for Staffing Policies in Long-Term Care Homes During and After the COVID-19 Pandemic." *Journal of the American Medical Directors Association* 21, no. 10: 1390–1. https://doi.org/10.1016/J.JAMDA.2020.07.036.

Edwards, Melissa. 2020. "Go Figure: What You May Not Know about Child Care in B.C." *BC Business*, 13 November 2020. https://www.bcbusiness.ca/What-you-may-not-know-about-child-care-in-BC.

Elson, Diane. 2010. "Gender and the Global Economic Crisis in Developing Countries: A Framework for Analysis." *Gender & Development* 18, no. 2: 201–12. https://doi.org/10.1080/13552074.2010.491321.

Epstein, Elizabeth, and Ashley Hurst. 2017. "Looking at the Positive Side of Moral Distress: Why It's a Problem." *Journal of Clinical Ethics* 28, no. 1: 37–41. https://pubmed.ncbi.nlm.nih.gov/28436927.

Esplen, Emily. 2009. *Gender and Care Overview Report*. Brighton: Institute for Development Studies. https://gsdrc.org/document-library/gender-and-care-overview-report.

Estabrooks, Carole A., Sharon E. Straus, Colleen M. Flood, Janice Keefe, Pat Armstrong, Gail J. Donner, Véronique Boscart, Francine Ducharme, James L. Silvius, and Michael C. Wolfson. 2020. "Restoring Trust: COVID-19 and the Future of Long-Term Care in Canada." *Facets* 5, no. 1: 651–91. https://doi.org/10.1139/FACETS-2020-0056.

Fawcett, Max. 2021. "Jason Kenney Government Teaches All the Wrong Lessons." *National Observer*, 1 April 2021. https://www.nationalobserver.com/2021/03/31/opinion/jason-kenney-government-teaches-all-wrong-lessons.

Fineman, Martha. 2001. "Contract and Care." *Chicago-Kent Law Review* 76, no. 3: 1403–40 https://scholarship.kentlaw.iit.edu/cklawreview/vol76/iss3/3.

Folbre, Nancy. 2008. "Reforming Care." *Politics and Society* 36, no. 3: 373–87. https://doi.org/10.1177/0032329208320567.

Folbre, Nancy, Leila Gautham, and Kristin Smith. 2021. "Essential Workers and Care Penalties in the United States." *Feminist Economics* 27, no. 1–2: 173–87. https://doi.org/10.1080/13545701.2020.1828602/SUPPL_FILE/RFEC_A_1828602_SM1133.PDF.

Foster, Victoria. 2020. "Women Are Leading Canada's Public Health Response to the COVID-19 Coronavirus Outbreak." *Forbes*, 14 April 2020. https://www.forbes.com/sites/victoriaforster/2020/04/14/women-are-leading-canadas-public-health-response-to-the-coronavirus-covid-19-outbreak/?sh=3a751d9464ae.

Gadermann, Anne C., Kimberly C. Thomson, Chris G. Richardson, Monique Gagné, Corey McAuliffe, Saima Hirani, and Emily Jenkins. 2021. "Examining the Impacts of the COVID-19 Pandemic on Family Mental Health in Canada: Findings from a National Cross-Sectional Study." *BMJ Open* 11, no. 1: e042871. https://doi.org/10.1136/BMJOPEN-2020-042871.

Gale, Nicola K., Gemma Heath, Elaine Cameron, Sabina Rashid, and Sabi Redwood. 2013. "Using the Framework Method for the Analysis of Qualitative Data in Multi-Disciplinary Health Research." *BMC Medical Research Methodology* 13, no. 1: 117. https://doi.org/10.1186/1471-2288-13-117.

Gilligan, Carol. 2016. "Reply to Critics." In *An Ethic of Care: Feminist and Interdisciplinary Perspectives*, edited by Mary Jean Larrabee, 207–14. New York: Routledge. https://doi.org/10.4324/9780203760192-26.

Gilligan, Carol, Janie Victoria Ward, and Jill Mclean Taylor, eds. 1988. *Mapping the Moral Domain: A Contribution of Women's Thinking to Psychological Theory and Education.* Harvard University Press.

Goldberg, Simon B., Sin U. Lam, Otto Simonsson, John Torous, and Shufang Sunid. 2022. "Mobile Phone-Based Interventions for Mental Health: A Systematic Meta-Review of 14 Meta-Analyses of Randomized Controlled Trials." *PLOS Digital Health* 1, no. 1: e0000002. https://doi.org/10.1371/JOURNAL.PDIG.0000002.

Government of BC. 2020. "Essential Services." Victoria: Government of BC. https://www2.gov.bc.ca/assets/gov/family-and-social-supports/covid-19/list_of_essential_services.pdf.

Government of Canada. 2020. "Fall Economic Statement 2020." Ottawa: Government of Canada. https://www.budget.gc.ca/fes-eea/2020/home-accueil-en.html.

– 2021. "Budget 2021: A Canada-Wide Early Learning and Child Care Plan." Ottawa: Government of Canada. https://www.canada.ca/en/department-finance/news/2021/04/budget-2021-a-canada-wide-early-learning-and-child-care-plan.html.

Gray, Benjamin. 2009. "The Emotional Labour of Nursing 1: Exploring the Concept." *Nursing Times* 105, no. 8: 26–9. https://europepmc.org/article/med/19331081.

Guest, Greg, Kathleen M. MacQueen, and Emily E. Namey. 2014. "Introduction to Applied Thematic Analysis." In *Applied Thematic Analysis*, edited by Greg Guest, Kathleen M. MacQueen, and Emily E. Namey, 3–20. Thousand Oaks: SAGE. https://doi.org/10.4135/9781483384436.

Guppy, Neil, Larissa Sakumoto, and Rima Wilkes. 2019. "Social Change and the Gendered Division of Household Labor in Canada." *Canadian Review of Sociology/Revue Canadienne de Sociologie* 56, no. 2: 178–203. https://doi.org/10.1111/CARS.12242.

Habermas, Jürgen. 1987. *The Theory of Communicative Action*, vol. 2, *Lifeworld and System: A Critique of Functionalist Reason*. Boston: Beacon Press.

Haeck, Catherine, and Simon Larose. 2022. "What is the Effect of School Closures on Learning in Canada? A Hypothesis Informed by International Data." *Canadian Journal of Public Health* 113: 36–43.

Halfon, Shani, and Rachel Langford. 2015. "Developing and Supporting a High Quality Child Care Workforce in Canada: What Are the Barriers to Change?" Ottawa: Canadian Centre for Policy Alternatives. https://www.policyalternatives.ca/sites/default/files/

uploads/publications/National Office/2015/09/OS120_Summer2015_
Workforce.pdf.

Harman, Sophie. 2016. "Ebola, Gender and Conspicuously Invisible
Women in Global Health Governance." *Third World Quarterly* 37, no. 3:
524–41. https://www.tandfonline.com/doi/abs/10.1080/01436597.
2015.1108827?journalCode=ctwq20.

– 2021. "Threat Not Solution: Gender, Global Health Security and
COVID-19." *International Affairs* 97, no. 3: 601–23. https://doi.
org/10.1093/IA/IIAB012.

Havaei, Farinaz, Ibrahim Abughori, Yue Mao, Sabina Staempfli,
Andy Ma, Maura MacPhee, Alison Phinney, et al. 2022. "The Impact
of Pandemic Management Strategies on Staff Mental Health, Work
Behaviours, and Resident Care in One Long-Term Care Facility in
British Columbia: A Mixed Method Study." *Journal of Long-Term
Care*, March, 71–87. https://doi.org/10.31389/JLTC.100

Hawke, Lisa, Peter Szatmari, Kristin Cleverley, Darren Courtney,
Amy Cheung, Aristotle Vioneskos, and Joanna Henderson. 2021.
"Youth in a Pandemic: A Longitudinal Examination of Youth Mental
Health and Substance Use Concerns during COVID-19." *BMJ Open* 11,
no. 10: e049209.

HEU. 2021. "Province Reverses Privatization of Cleaning and Dietary
Work in B.C. Hospitals." Vancouver: Hospital Employees' Union.
https://www.heu.org/news/media-release/province-reverses-privatization-
cleaning-and-dietary-work-bc-hospitals.

– 2022. "Poll: Two Years into Pandemic, One in Three Health Care
Workers Likely to Quit." Vancouver: Hospital Employees' Union.
https://www.heu.org/news/media-release/poll-two-years-pandemic-one-
three-health-care-workers-likely-quit.

Hjálmsdóttir, Andrea, Valgerður S. Bjarnadóttir, and Minningasjóður
Eðvarðs Sigurðssonar. 2021. "'I Have Turned into a Foreman Here
at Home': Families and Work-Life Balance in Times of COVID-19
in a Gender Equality Paradise." *Gender, Work & Organization* 28,
no. 1: 268–83. https://doi.org/10.1111/GWAO.12552.

Hossain, Fahmida. 2021. "Moral Distress among Healthcare Providers
and Mistrust among Patients during COVID-19 in Bangladesh."
Developing World Bioethics 21, no. 4: 187–92. https://doi.org/10.1111/
DEWB.12291.

Hrymak, Haley, and Kim Hawkins. 2021. "Why Can't Everyone Just
Get Along? How BC's Family Law System Puts Survivors in Danger."
Vancouver: Rise Women's Legal Centre. https://womenslegalcentre.ca/

wp-content/uploads/2021/01/Why-Cant-Everyone-Just-Get-Along-Rise-Womens-Legal-January2021.pdf.

Isenbarger, Lynn, and Michalinos Zembylas. 2006. "The Emotional Labour of Caring in Teaching." *Teaching and Teacher Education* 22, no. 1: 120–34. https://doi.org/10.1016/j.tate.2005.07.002.

Ismail, Aziah, Nor Shafrin Ahmad, and Rahimi Che Aman. 2021. "Gender of Transformational School Principals and Teachers' Innovative Behavior." *International Journal of Evaluation and Research in Education* 10, no. 3: 747–52. http://doi.org/10.11591/ijere.v10i3.21448.

Ivanova, Iglika, Shannon Daub, and Anastasia French. 2022. "Working for a Living Wage: Making Paid Work Meet Basic Family Needs in Metro Vancouver." Vancouver: BC Office, Canadian Centre for Policy Alternatives. https://policyalternatives.ca/sites/default/files/uploads/publications/BC%20Office/2022/11/CCPA-BC-Living-Wage-Update-2022-final.pdf.

Jameton, A. 1993. "Dilemmas of Moral Distress: Moral Responsibility and Nursing Practice." *Clinical Issues in Perinatal and Women's Health Nursing* 4, no. 4: 542–51. https://repository.library.georgetown.edu/handle/10822/860982.

Jones, Yemisi, Vanessa Durand, Kayce Morton, Mary Ottolini, Erin Shaughnessy, Nancy D. Spector, and Jennifer O'Toole. 2020. "Collateral Damage: How COVID-19 Is Adversely Impacting Women Physicians." *Journal of Hospital Medicine* 15, no. 8: 507–9. https://doi.org/10.12788/jhm.3470.

Kofman, Yasmin B., and Dana Rose Garfin. 2020. "Home Is Not Always a Haven: The Domestic Violence Crisis amid the COVID-19 Pandemic." *Psychological Trauma: Theory, Research, Practice, and Policy* 12, no. S1: S199–201. https://doi.org/10.1037/TRA0000866.

Krase, Kathryn, Leina Luzuriaga, Donna Wang, Andrew Schoolnik, Latoya Attis, and Petra Brown. 2021. "Exploring the Impact of Gender on Challenges and Coping during the COVID-19 Pandemic." *International Journal of Sociology and Social Policy* 42, no. 11: 1–12.

Kurt, Osman, Seuleyman Erhane Deveci, and Ayse Ferdane Oguzoncul. 2020. "Levels of Anxiety and Depression Related to COVID-19 among Physicians: An Online Cross-Sectional Study from Turkey." *Annals of Clinical and Analytical Medicine* 11, suppl. 3: S288–93. https://doi.org/10.4328/acam.20206.

Lake, Eileen T., Aliza M. Narva, Sara Holland, Jessica G. Smith, Emily Cramer, Kathleen E. Fitzpatrick Rosenbaum, Rachel French, Rebecca R.S. Clark, and Jeannette A. Rogowski. 2022. "Hospital Nurses' Moral

Distress and Mental Health during COVID-19." *Journal of Advanced Nursing* 78, no. 3: 799–809. https://doi.org/10.1111/JAN.15013.

Larochelle-Côté, Sébastien, and Sharanjit Uppal. 2020. "The Social and Economic Concerns of Immigrants during the COVID-19 Pandemic." Ottawa: Statistics Canada. https://www150.statcan.gc.ca/n1/pub/45-28-0001/2020001/article/00012-eng.htm.

Larrabee, Mary Jeanne, ed. 2016. *An Ethic of Care: Feminist and Interdisciplinary Perspectives.* New York: Routledge. https://doi.org/10.4324/9780203760192.

Lightman, Naomi. 2021. "Caring during the COVID-19 Crisis: Intersectional Exclusion of Immigrant Women Health Care Aides in Canadian Long-Term Care." *Health & Social Care in the Community* 30, no. 4: e1343–51. https://doi.org/10.1111/HSC.13541.

Lizana, Pablo A., Gustavo Vega-Fernandez, Alejandro Gomez-Bruton, Bárbara Leyton, and Lydia Lera. 2021. "Impact of the COVID-19 Pandemic on Teacher Quality of Life: A Longitudinal Study from before and during the Health Crisis." *International Journal of Environmental Research and Public Health* 18, no. 7: 3764. https://doi.org/10.3390/ijerph18073764.

Lokot, Michelle, Amiya Bhatia, Shirin Heidari, and Amber Peterman. 2021. "The Pitfalls of Modelling the Effects of COVID-19 on Gender-Based Violence: Lessons Learnt and Ways Forward." *BMJ Global Health* 6, no. 5: e005739. https://doi.org/10.1136/BMJGH-2021-005739.

Lovell, Brenda, Raymond Lee, and Céleste Brotheridge. 2009. "Gender Differences in the Application of Communication Skills, Emotional Labor, Stress-coping, and Well-being among Physicians." *International Journal of Medicine* 2, no. 3: 273–8. https://go.gale.com/ps/i.do?id=GALE%7CA209537187&sid=googleScholar&v=2.1&it=r&link access=abs&issn=17914000&p=HRCA&sw=w&userGroupName=anon%7Efb175672

MABC. 2022. "Midwives Deliver." Vancouver: Midwives Association of BC. https://www.bcmidwives.com.

Macdonald, David. 2018. *Child Care Deserts in Canada.* Ottawa: Canadian Centre for Policy Alternatives. https://www.policyalternatives.ca/publications/reports/child-care-deserts-canada.

Macdonald, David, and Martha Friendly. 2017. *Time Out: Childcare Fees in Canada in 2017.* Canadian Centre for Policy Alternatives. https://policyalternatives.ca/sites/default/files/uploads/publications/National%20Office/2017/12/Time%20Out.pdf.

– 2021. *Sounding the Alarm*. Ottawa: Canadian Centre for Policy Alternatives. https://www.policyalternatives.ca/TheAlarm.

MacDonald, Margaret, and Cher Hill. 2022. "The Educational Impact of the Covid-19 Rapid Response on Teachers, Students, and Families: Insights from British Columbia, Canada." *Prospects* 51, no. 4: 627–41.

MacPhee, Maura, V. Susan Dahinten, and Farinaz Havaei. 2017. "The Impact of Heavy Perceived Nurse Workloads on Patient and Nurse Outcomes." *Administrative Sciences* 7, no. 1: 7. https://doi.org/10.3390/ADMSCI7010007.

Matiz, Alessio, Franco Fabbro, Andrea Paschetto, Daminio Cantone, Anselmo Paolone, and Cristiano Crescentini. 2020. "Positive Impact of Mindfulness Meditation on Mental Health of Female Teachers during the COVID-19 Outbreak in Italy." *International Journal of Environmental Research and Public Health* 17, no. 18: 6450.

Maunder, Robert G. 2009. "Was SARS a Mental Health Catastrophe?" *General Hospital Psychiatry* 31, no. 4: 316–17. https://doi.org/10.1016/J.GENHOSPPSYCH.2009.04.004.

McCloskey, Rose, Cindy Donovan, and Alicia Donovan. 2017. "Linking Incidents in Long-Term Care Facilities to Worker Activities." *Workplace Health and Safety* 65, no. 10: 457–66. https://doi.org/10.1177/2165079916680366.

McIntosh, Ian, and Sharon Wright. 2019. "Exploring What the Notion of 'Lived Experience' Offers for Social Policy Analysis." *Journal of Social Policy* 48, no. 3: 449–67. https://doi.org/10.1017/S0047279418000570.

McLaren, Helen Jaqueline, Karen Rosalind Wong, Kieu Nga Nguyen, and Komalee Nadeeka Damayanthi Mahamadachchi. 2020. "Covid-19 and Women's Triple Burden: Vignettes from Sri Lanka, Malaysia, Vietnam and Australia." *Social Sciences* 9, no. 5: 87. https://doi.org/10.3390/SOCSCI9050087.

McPhail, Beverly A. 2003. "A Feminist Policy Analysis Framework." *Social Policy Journal* 2, no. 3: 39–61. https://doi.org/10.1300/J185v02n02_04.

Mejia, Cynthia, Rebecca Pittman, Jenna M.D. Beltramo, Kristin Horan, Amanda Grinley, and Mindy K. Shoss. 2021. "Stigma & Dirty Work: In-Group and Out-Group Perceptions of Essential Service Workers during COVID-19." *International Journal of Hospitality Management* 93 (February): 102772. https://doi.org/10.1016/J.IJHM.2020.102772.

Milne, Kendra. 2016. "High Stakes: The Impacts of Child Care on the
    Human Rights of Women and Children." Vancouver: West Coast
    Women's Legal Education and Action Fund. https://www.westcoastleaf.
    org/wp-content/uploads/2016/07/High-Stakes-low-res-for-web.pdf.

Monteblanco, Adelle Dora. 2021. "The COVID-19 Pandemic: A Focusing
    Event to Promote Community Midwifery Policies in the United States."
    Social Sciences & Humanities Open 3, no. 1: 100104. https://doi.
    org/10.1016/J.SSAHO.2020.100104.

Mooi-Reci, Irma, and Barbara J. Risman. 2021. "The Gendered Impacts
    of COVID-19: Lessons and Reflections." Gender & Society 35, no. 2:
    161–7. https://doi.org/10.1177/08912432211001305.

Morgan, Rosemary, Asha George, Sarah Ssali, Kate Hawkins,
    Sassy Molyneux, and Sally Theobald. 2016. "How to Do (or Not
    to Do) … Gender Analysis in Health Systems Research." Health
    Policy and Planning 31, no. 8: 1069–78. https://doi.org/10.1093/
    heapol/czw037.

Morgan, Rosemary, Heang-Lee Tan, Niki Oveisi, Christina Memmott,
    Alexander Korzuchowski, Kate Hawkins, and Julia Smith. 2022.
    "Women Healthcare Workers' Experiences during COVID-19 and
    Other Crises: A Scoping Review." International Journal of Nursing
    Studies Advances 4 (December): 100066. https://doi.org/10.1016/J.
    IJNSA.2022.100066.

Morley, Georgina, Denise Sese, Prabalini Rajendram, and Cristie Cole
    Horsburgh. 2020. "Addressing Caregiver Moral Distress during the
    COVID-19 Pandemic." Cleveland Clinic Journal of Medicine, 89,
    no. 11:1–5. https://doi.org/10.3949/CCJM.87A.CCC047.

Mousa, Mariam, Jacqueline Boyle, Helen Skouteris, Alexandra K.
    Mullins, Graeme Currie, Kathleen Riach, and Helena J. Teede. 2021.
    "Advancing Women in Healthcare Leadership: A Systematic Review
    and Meta-Synthesis of Multi-Sector Evidence on Organisational
    Interventions." EClinicalMedicine 39 (September): 101084. https://doi.
    org/10.1016/J.ECLINM.2021.101084.

Murphy, Patricia Aikins. 2020. "Midwifery in the Time of COVID-19."
    Journal of Midwifery & Women's Health 65, no. 3: 299–300. https://
    doi.org/10.1111/JMWH.13121.

Nethery, Elizabeth, Laura Schummers, Audrey Levine, Aaron B.
    Caughey, Vivienne Souter, and Wendy Gordon. 2021. "Birth Outcomes
    for Planned Home and Licensed Freestanding Birth Center Births in
    Washington State." Obstetrics and Gynecology 138, no. 5: 693–702.
    https://doi.org/10.1097/AOG.0000000000004578.

O'Connell, Christopher B. 2015. "Gender and the Experience of Moral Distress in Critical Care Nurses." *Nursing Ethics* 22, no.1: 32–42. https://doi.org/10.1177/0969733013513216.

Office of the Premier – Province of British Columbia. 2018. "Premier John Horgan Appoints Mitzi Dean as Parliamentary Secretary for Gender Equity." News release, 15 February 2018. https://news.gov. bc.ca/releases/2018PREM0023-000215.

Office of the Seniors Advocate. 2020. *A Billion Reasons to Care: A Funding Review of Contracted Long-Term Care in B.C.* Victoria: Seniors Advocate of BC. https://www.seniorsadvocatebc.ca/app/uploads/ sites/4/2020/02/ABillionReasonsToCare.pdf.

– 2021. *Review of COVID-19 Outbreaks in Care Homes in British Columbia – Seniors Advocate.* Victoria: Seniors Advocate of BC. https:// www.seniorsadvocatebc.ca/osa-reports/covid-outbreak-review-report.

Oliu-Barton, Miquel, Bary S.R. Pradelski, Philippe Aghion, Patrick Artus, Ilona Kickbusch, Jeffrey V. Lazarus, Devi Sridhar, and Samantha Vanderslott. 2021. "SARS-COV-2 Elimination, Not Mitigation, Creates Best Outcomes for Health, the Economy, and Civil Liberties." *The Lancet* 397, no. 10291: 2234–6. https://doi.org/10.1016/ S0140-6736(21)00978-8/attachment/5b160506-ca75-43fb-9d8b- cf2d1e4b8713/mmc2.pdf.

Oxfam Canada. 2020. "Unpaid Care Work Caused by COVID-19." Ottawa: Oxfam Canada. https://www.oxfam.ca/news/71-per-cent-of- canadian-women-feeling-more-anxious-depressed-isolated-overworked- or-ill-because-of-increased-unpaid-care-work-caused-by-covid-19- oxfam-survey.

Paterson, Stephanie. 2010. "What's the Problem with Gender-Based Analysis? Gender Mainstreaming Policy and Practice in Canada." *Canadian Public Administration* 53, no. 3: 395–416. https://doi. org/10.1111/j.1754-7121.2010.00134.x.

Pauly, Bernadette M., Colleen Varcoe, and Jan Storch. 2012. "Framing the Issues: Moral Distress in Health Care." *HEC Forum: An Interdisciplinary Journal on Hospitals' Ethical and Legal Issues* 24, no. 1: 1–11. https://doi.org/10.1007/S10730-012-9176-Y.

Pijl-Zieber, Em, Brad Hagen, Chris Armstrong-Esther, Barry Hall, Lindsay Akins, and Michael Stingl. 2008. "Moral Distress: An Emerging Problem for Nurses in Long-Term Care?" *Quality in Ageing* 9, no. 2: 39–48. https://doi.org/10.1108/14717794200800013.

Pinquart, Martin, and Silvia Sörensen. 2006. "Gender Differences in Caregiver Stressors, Social Resources, and Health: An Updated

Meta-Analysis." *Journals of Gerontology* 61, no. 1: P33–45. https://doi. org/10.1093/GERONB/61.1.P33.

Poghosyan, Lusine, Linda H. Aiken, and Douglas Sloane. 2009. "Factor Structure of the Maslach Burnout Inventory: An Analysis of Data from Large-Scale Cross-Sectional Surveys of Nurses from Eight Countries." *International Journal of Nursing Studies* 46, no. 7: 894–902. https:// doi.org/10.1016/j.ijnurstu.2009.03.004.

Porter, Catherine. 2020. "The Top Doctor Who Aced the Coronavirus Test." *New York Times*, 5 June 2020. https://www.nytimes.com/2020/06/ 05/world/canada/bonnie-henry-british-columbia-coronavirus.html.

Powell, Alana, Rachel Langford, Patrizia Albanese, Susan Prentice, and Kate Bezanson. 2020. "Who Cares for Carers? How Discursive Constructions of Care Work Marginalized Early Childhood Educators in Ontario's 2018 Provincial Election." *Contemporary Issues in Early Childhood* 21, no. 2: 153–64. https://doi. org/10.1177/1463949120928433.

Qian, Yue, and Sylvia Fuller. 2020. "COVID-19 and the Gender Employment Gap among Parents of Young Children." *Canadian Public Policy* 46, suppl. 2: S89–101. https://doi.org/10.3138/CPP.2020-077.

Rai, Shirin, and Georgina Waylen. 2013. *New Frontiers in Feminist Political Economy*. London: Taylor and Francis. https://doi.org/ 10.4324/9781315884745.

Rudrum, Sarah. 2021. "Pregnancy during the Global COVID-19 Pandemic: Canadian Experiences of Care." *Frontiers in Sociology* 6 (February): 2. https://doi.org/10.3389/FSOC.2021.611324.

Safecare BC. 2017. "New Strategy Is Needed to Address Shortage of Continuing Care Workers – Safecare BC." Vancouver: Safecare BC. https://www.safecarebc.ca/2017/05/16/media-release-new-strategy- needed-address-shortage-continuing-care-workers.

Sandall, Jane, Hora Soltani, Simon Gates, Andrew Shennan, and Declan Devane. 2016. "Midwife-Led Continuity Models versus Other Models of Care for Childbearing Women." *Cochrane Database of Systematic Reviews* 4, no. 4: CD004667. https://doi.org/10.1002/14651858. CD004667.PUB5.

Schwarzenbach, Sibyl. 1996. "On Civic Friendship." *Ethics* 107, no. 1: 97–128. https://www.jstor.org/stable/2382245?seq=1.

Sese, Denise, Mahwish U. Ahmad, and Prabalini Rajendram. 2020. "Ethical Considerations during the COVID-19 Pandemic." *Cleveland Clinic Journal of Medicine* (June): 1–6. https://doi.org/10.3949/ CCJM.87A.CCC038.

Seyd, Jane. 2020. "Lynn Valley Care Home Resident Canada's First Coronavirus Death." *North Shore News*, 9 March 2020. https://www.nsnews.com/local-news/lynn-valley-care-home-resident-canadas-first-coronavirus-death-3118557.

Shore, Randy. 2020. "Anti-Chinese Racism Is Canada's 'Shadow Pandemic,' Say Researchers." *Vancouver Sun*, 22 June 2020. https://vancouversun.com/news/anti-chinese-racism-is-canadas-shadow-pandemic-say-researchers.

Shrma, Lokpriy, and Julia Smith. 2021. "COVID-19's Effects on the Healthcare and Social Assistance Workforce in Canada: Gendered Employment Loss and Wage Inequality 2020–2021." Burnaby: Simon Fraser University. https://www.genderandcovid-19.org/wp-content/uploads/2021/11/PAC00490_Gender-and-Covid-19-Canadian-Healthcare.pdf.

Silverio-Murillo, Adan, Jose Roberto Balmori de la Miyar, and Lauren Hoehn-Velasco. 2020. "Families under Confinement: COVID-19, Domestic Violence, and Alcohol Consumption." *SSRN Electronic Journal* (September). https://doi.org/10.2139/ssrn.3688384.

Smith, Julia. 2019. "Overcoming the 'Tyranny of the Urgent': Integrating Gender into Disease Outbreak Preparedness and Response." *Gender and Development* 27, no. 2: 355–69. https://doi.org/10.1080/13552074.2019.1615288.

Smith-Johnson, Tanya, Deja Ostrowski, Jen Jenkins, Darlene Ewan, Kathleen Algire, Angelina Mercado, and Healthy Mothers Healthy Babies. 2020. *Building Bridges, Not Walking on Backs: A Feminist Economic Recovery Plan for COVID-19.* Honolulu: Hawai'i State Commission on the Status of Women. https://humanservices.hawaii.gov/wp-content/uploads/2020/04/4.13.20-Final-Cover-D2-Feminist-Economic-Recovery-D1.pdf.

Sokal, Laura, Lesley G. Eblie Trudel, and Jeff C. Babb. 2020. "Supporting Teachers in Times of Change: The Job Demands-Resources Model and Teacher Burnout During the COVID-19 Pandemic." *International Journal of Contemporary Education* 3, no. 2: 67–74.

Sproule, Roxanne, and Alana Prochuk. 2020. "BC Gender Equality Report Card 2019/2020." Vancouver: West Coast Leaf. https://www.westcoastleaf.org/our-publications/report-card-2019-2020.

Statistics Canada. 2018. "Time Use: Total Work Burden, Unpaid Work, and Leisure." Ottawa: Government of Canada. https://www150.statcan.gc.ca/n1/pub/89-503-x/2015001/article/54931-eng.htm.

– 2020a. "The Daily – Impacts of COVID-19 on Canadians: First Results from Crowdsourcing." Ottawa: Government of Canada. https://www150.statcan.gc.ca/n1/daily-quotidien/200423/dq200423a-eng.htm.

– 2020b. "Impacts of COVID-19 on Immigrants and People Designated as Visible Minorities." Ottawa: Government of Canada. https://www150.statcan.gc.ca/n1/pub/11-631-x/2020004/s6-eng.htm.

– 2021. "The Daily – Births, 2020." Ottawa: Government of Canada. https://www150.statcan.gc.ca/n1/daily-quotidien/210928/dq210928d-eng.htm.

Stelnicki, Andrea M., R. Nicholas Carleton, and Carol Reichert. 2020. "Nurses' Mental Health and Well-Being: COVID-19 Impacts." *Canadian Journal of Nursing Research / Revue canadienne de recherche en sciences infirmières* 52, no. 3: 237–9. https://doi.org/10.1177/0844562120931623.

Stoll, Kathrin, and Jocelyn Gallagher. 2019. "A Survey of Burnout and Intentions to Leave the Profession among Western Canadian Midwives." *Women and Birth: Journal of the Australian College of Midwives* 32, no. 4: e441–9. https://doi.org/10.1016/J.WOMBI.2018.10.002.

Sultana, Anjum, and Carmina Ravanera. 2020. *A Feminist Economic Recovery Plan for Canada: Making the Economy Work for Everyone.* Toronto: YWCA. https://www.feministrecovery.ca.

Tallis, Vicci. 2012. *Feminisms, HIV and AIDS.* London: Palgrave Macmillan. https://doi.org/10.1057/9781137005793_3.

Tricco, Andrea C., Ivy Bourgeault, Ainsley Moore, Eva Grunfeld, Nazia Peer, and Sharon E. Straus. 2021. "Advancing Gender Equity in Medicine." *CMAJ* 193, no. 7: E244–50. https://doi.org/10.1503/CMAJ.200951.

Trix, Frances, and Carolyn Psenka. 2016. "Exploring the Color of Glass: Letters of Recommendation for Female and Male Medical Faculty." *Discourse and Society* 14, no. 2: 191–220. https://doi.org/10.1177/0957926503014002277.

Tronto, Joan. 2013. *Caring Democracy.* New York: NYU Press. https://nyupress.org/9780814782781/caring-democracy.

Turrentine, Florence E., Caitlin N. Dreisbach, Amanda R. St Ivany, John B. Hanks, and Anneke T. Schroen. 2019. "Influence of Gender on Surgical Residency Applicants' Recommendation Letters." *Journal of the American College of Surgeons* 228, no. 4: 356–65e3. https://doi.org/10.1016/J.JAMCOLLSURG.2018.12.020.

UNDP. 2022. "COVID-19 Global Gender Response Tracker." New York: United Nations Development Programme. https://data.undp.org/ gendertracker.

UN Women. 2021. *Beyond COVID-19: A Feminist Plan for Sustainability and Social Justice*. New York: UN Women. https://www.unwomen.org/ en/digital-library/publications/2021/09/ beyond-covid-19-a-feminist-plan-for-sustainability-and-social-justice.

Uppal, Sharanjit, and Katherine Savage. 2021. "Child Care Workers in Canada." Ottawa: Statistics Canada. https://www150.statcan.gc.ca/n1/ pub/75-006-x/2021001/article/00005-eng.htm.

van Daalen, Kim Robin, Csongor Bajnoczki, Maisoon Chowdhury, Sara Dada, Parnian Khorsand, Anna Socha, Arush Lal, et al. 2020. "Symptoms of a Broken System: The Gender Gaps in COVID-19 Decision-Making." *BMJ Global Health* 5, no. 10: e003549. https://doi. org/10.1136/BMJGH-2020-003549.

Vollans, Andrea. 2010. "Court-Related Abuse and Harassment." Vancouver: YWCA Vancouver. https://ywcavan.org/sites/default/files/ assets/media/file/2021-01%20/Court-Related%20Abuse%20and%20 Harassment.pdf.

Vosko, J.F., and L.F. Zukewich. 2003. "The Gender of Precarious Employment in Canada." *Industrial Relations* 58, no. 3: 454–82. https://doi.org/10.7202/007495ar.

Wallace, Rebecca, and Elizabeth Goodyear-Grant. 2020. "News Coverage of Child Care during COVID-19: Where Are Women and Gender?" *Politics and Gender* 16, no. 4: 1123–30. https://doi.org/10.1017/ S1743923X20000598.

Warren, Karen, and Duane Cady. 1994. "Feminism and Peace: Seeing Connections." *Hypatia* 9 no. 2: 4–20. https://www.jstor.org/ stable/3810167.

Watson, Amanda. 2020. *The Juggling Mother – Coming Undone in the Age of Anxiety*. Vancouver: UBC Press. https://www.ubcpress.ca/ the-juggling-mother.

Wenham, Clare, and Asha Herten-Crabb. 2021. "It's a Distraction to Focus on the Success of Individual Women Leaders during Covid." *Kings College London News Centre*, 11 May 2021. https://www.kcl. ac.uk/news/individual-women-leaders-covid.

Wenham, Clare, Julia Smith, and Rosemary Morgan. 2020. "COVID-19: The Gendered Impacts of the Outbreak." *The Lancet* 395, no. 10227: 846–8. https://www.thelancet.com/journals/lancet/article/PIIS0140- 6736(20)30526-2/fulltext.

WGH. 2020. "A High Level Digital Summit: Women in Global Health Security – Foreign Policy." *Foreign Policy*, 17 September 2020. https://foreignpolicy.com/events/women-in-global-health.

Women and Gender Equality Canada. 2022. "Gender-Based Analysis Plus (GBA+)." Ottawa: Government of Canada. https://women-gender-equality.canada.ca/en/gender-based-analysis-plus.html.

Yakubovich, Alexa R., and Krys Maki. 2021. "Preventing Gender-Based Homelessness in Canada during the COVID-19 Pandemic and Beyond: The Need to Account for Violence Against Women." *Violence Against Women* 28, no. 10: 2587–699. https://doi.org/10.1177/10778012211034202.

Yarrow, Emily, and Victoria Pagan. 2020. "Reflections on Front-Line Medical Work during COVID-19 and the Embodiment of Risk." *Gender, Work & Organization* 28, no. S1: 89–100. https://doi.org/10.1111/gwao.12505.

Index

daycare. *See* child care

deaths, from COVID-19, 6;
  in long-term care facilities,
  31–2, 44

decision-making: childcare
  educators and, 136, 138, 157,
  160; long-term care workers and,
  47–8; midwives and, 122–5;
  nurses and, 89–1, 160; physicians
  and, 149, 150; teachers and,
  74–5, 160; women's involvement
  into, 28, 159, 160

depression: long-term care workers
  and, 44; nurses and, 78, 84, 85,
  88–9; physicians and, 147;
  women and, 5, 24, 25, 105.
  See also mental health and
  mental wellness

D'Ignazio, Catherine, and Lauren
  Klein, 28–9

discrimination: Asian Canadians
  and, 47; gender, 14; long-term
  care workers and, 47

doctors. *See* physicians

Doctors of BC, 146

domestic violence, 5. *See also*
  intimate partner violence (IPV)

double shift, 141, 145, 159

Early Childhood Educators of BC
  (ECEBC), 128

earnings. *See* income; wages

Ebola outbreak (2014–16), 3–4, 26

education: in Alberta, 55; early
  childhood, 128; interruptions in,
  156; mothers' responsibility for
  children's, 102–3; school closures, 53, 61, 104–5, 128. *See
  also* online learning; professional
  development

elder care: childcare educators and,
  131–2; long-term care workers
  and, 37; physicians and 148,
  151; teachers and, 62–3

emergency rooms, 142

emotional labour, 22, 96, 157;
  childcare educators and, 130;
  long-term care workers and, 36,
  157; midwives and, 113, 157;
  mothers and, 22, 96; physicians
  and, 151; school leaders and,
  58–9; teachers and, 59–60, 75,
  157; women and, 21–2

Employment Insurance (EI),
  99, 137

essential status, 20, 22–4, 157–8;
  childcare educators and, 132–4,
  138; as defined by Government
  of British Columbia, 24;
  long-term care workers and,
  38–42; midwives and, 115–18;
  mothers and, 103–5; nurses and,
  82–3; physicians and, 145–7;
  teachers and, 63–6

essential workers: child care
  for, 95, 104, 127, 128, 138;
  incompatibility of childcare
  hours and shift work for, 80,
  144; risk of COVID-19
  infection, 23

"ethic of rights," 12–13

family courts: closures of, 108–9

family responsibilities: gendered
  division of, 100–1. *See also* child
  care; elder care

fathers, care responsibilities and,
  95, 97, 100–1

federal government: cash transfers
  to parents, 96; "feminist"

supports and, 69; public health
protocols and, 56–7; risk of
COVID-19 infection, 63.
See also teachers
self-care: midwives and, 121;
mothers and, 106–7; nurses and,
86; teachers and, 69
sexism, 150
shift work: child care and, 114,
115, 144
sick leave benefits: childcare
educators and, 137; long-term-
care sector and, 41, 51; midwives
and, 118, 120–1; teachers and, 64
Simon Fraser University, ethical
approval for research, 16
single-site order, 32, 33
soft skills, in teaching, 71
staffing shortages: in long-term-care
facilities, 32, 33–5; in nursing,
78, 86; of substitute teachers,
64–5
stigma: long-term-care workers
and, 38–9; nurses and, 83
stress, 158; childcare educators
and, 134; moral distress and, 26;
mothers and, 105–6; physicians
and, 147–8; school leaders and
principals and, 58; teachers
and, 59, 68, 69; women and, 25
students: online learning and, 65–6,
102; teachers supporting, 59
substance use, 85–6, 159
support networks: for newcomer
childcare educators, 131; for
teachers, 61–2. *See also* peer
support networks

teachers, 53–76, 154; appreciation
and acknowledgment, 66, 75;
balancing child care and work

responsibilities, 60–1, 64, 68, 75;
burnout and, 66–7, 69, 75;
career aspirations and, 70–2, 73;
decision-making and, 74–5, 160;
effects of pandemic on, 53–4;
elder care and, 62–3; emotional
labour and, 59–60, 75, 157; as
essential, 63–6; further education
and qualifications, 71–2, 159;
guilt and, 68; increased unpaid
workloads, 60, 72–3; job
satisfaction and, 69; leadership
and, 70–2, 72–3; mental health
and wellness, 54, 66–7, 75;
mental health supports, 69;
moral distress and, 67–9; online
teaching and, 61, 65–6;
percentage identifying as women,
54; power and, 70–5; quadruple
burden and, 55–63; recommendations for improvements, 75–6;
research participants, 54; risk of
COVID-19 infection and, 63, 65;
self-care and, 69; shortage of
substitute, 64–5; sick leave and,
64; support networks and, 61–2;
vaccination priority and, 63–4,
157; working from home, 73–4
teaching, gendered nature of, 54
technology, for online learning, 102
therapy. *See* counselling and therapy
"time cultures," 21
touch: childcare educators and,
135; midwives and, 119
toxic drugs: deaths in British
Columbia, 7; nurses' workloads
and, 79
triple burden, 20, 21, 101
Trudeau, Justin, 23, 24
trust: decision-making and, 89–90;
long-term-care staff and, 50